*FAST*ANSWERS
Fasting Plans for Specific Prayer Needs

Beyr Reyes

Fast Answers: Fasting Plans for Specific Prayer Needs
Beyr Reyes
Copyright @ 2012 ShadeTree Publishing, LLC
Print ISBN: 978-1-937331-49-8
e-Book ISBN: 978-1-937331-50-4
Cover art by Josh Hickey

Throughout this book, brackets [ ] represent the author's addition and are not part of the quoted scripture.

Scripture quotations marked KJV are taken from the Holy Bible, King James Version, 1768 edition, which is in the public domain.

Scripture quotations marked NIV are taken from the Holy Bible, New International Version®, NIV®. Copyright © 1973, 1978, 1984, 2011 by Biblica US, Inc®. Used by permission.

Scripture quotations marked NKJV are taken from the Holy Bible, New King James Version, copyright © 1982 by Thomas Nelson, Inc. All rights reserved. Used by permission.

Note from Author: The word *unforgiveness* is not in the dictionary; however, it is a very real thing. As such, this word is used throughout this book to mean the act of not forgiving.

All rights reserved. This book is protected by copyright. No part of this book may be reproduced or transmitted in any form or by any means, electronic or mechanical, including photocopying, recording, or by any information storage and retrieval system, without permission in writing from the publisher.

The purpose of this book is to educate and enlighten. This book is sold with the understanding that the author and publisher are not engaged in rendering counseling, albeit it professional or lay, to the reader or anyone else. The author and publisher shall have neither liability nor responsibility to any person or entity with respect to any loss or damage caused, or alleged to have been caused, directly or indirectly, by the information contained in this book.

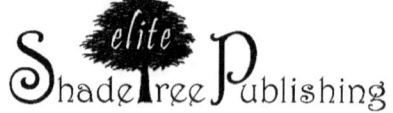

Visit our Web site at www.ShadeTreePublishing.com

I dedicate this book to all the readers who take fasting seriously.

Table of Contents

HOW TO USE THIS BOOK 1
INTRODUCTION 3
   WHAT IS A FAST? 5
   WHEN TO FAST 6
   WARNINGS ABOUT FASTING 7

WHEN YOU'VE BEEN HURT BY OTHERS 9
   WHEN YOU'VE LOST A LOVED ONE 11
   WHEN YOU'VE BEEN BETRAYED 19
   WHEN YOU'VE BEEN CHEATED ON 27
   WHEN YOU'VE BEEN STOLEN FROM 37
   WHEN YOU'VE BEEN LIED ABOUT OR LIED TO 45
   WHEN YOU'VE BEEN FORSAKEN 53

WHEN YOU'VE HURT OTHERS 61
   WHEN YOU'VE BETRAYED SOMEONE 63
   WHEN YOU'VE COMMITTED ADULTERY 71
   WHEN YOU NEED FORGIVENESS 79
   WHEN YOU'VE STOLEN FROM SOMEONE 87
   WHEN YOU'VE LIED 95
   WHEN YOU'VE FORSAKEN SOMEONE 103

WHEN YOU NEED ANSWERS AND DIRECTION 111
   WHEN YOU NEED A WORD FROM GOD 113
   WHEN YOU NEED A NEW MINDSET AND WAY OF THINKING 121
   WHEN YOU NEED CONFIRMATION 129
   WHEN YOU WANT GOD'S WILL FOR YOUR LIFE 137

OTHER IDEAS FOR FASTING 145
   SCRIPTURE FAST 147
   GROUPS OR TYPES OF PEOPLE 147
   TO ACCOMPLISH SOMETHING 148
   WHEN YOU DON'T KNOW THE REASON 149

ABOUT THE AUTHOR 151
NOTES 155

Fast Answers by Beyr Reyes

HOW TO USE THIS BOOK

This entire book was written during a forty-day fast. Many times, I would struggle with what to write, and God would come to my rescue. He punctuated some of the Fasting Plans with circumstances to give me a fresh perspective of feelings involved. For example, halfway through the two days when I wrote about losing a loved one, our former children's pastor died unexpectedly. While finishing the devotion, all I could think about were his young widow and three kids.

You may be asking whether the world needs another book about fasting. My answer is yes, because this book is different. Other books tell you why to fast or explain the importance thereof. Many times after reading these books, I would be so excited to start a fast, but then quickly realized that I didn't know how or where to begin.

This book isn't about fast answers (as in quick ones). It's about fast answers (as in seeking God ones). The goal for this book is to help people get answers and resolve problems by drawing closer to God through fasting.

This book is not meant to be read from cover to cover. Instead, use it as a tool for fasting.

Fast Answers is divided into the following units. (Depending on what your need is, navigate to that particular unit.)

- Introduction and background for fasting
- Fasting Plans for when you've been hurt by someone
- Fasting Plans for when you've hurt someone
- Fasting Plans for when you need answers and direction
- Various other ideas for fasting

The Fasting Plans address specific circumstances commonly associated with the theme of its unit. For example, within the "When You've Been Hurt by Others" unit, you will find Fasting

Fast Answers by Beyr Reyes

Plans dealing with betrayal, loss of a loved one, adultery, etc. Find the situation that best describes yours.

After you decide what you will be fasting about, decide how many days you will fast. The Fasting Plans come in one-, three-, and seven-day varieties. Choose the timing that best fits your need. For example, a scheduled fast might be better if it were seven days, whereas sometimes, in urgent needs, only one day is available.

Each Fasting Plan consists of a:

- Basic introduction
- Proclamation (addresses the purpose of the fast)
- Scripture for the day
- Question for the day
- Prayer for the day

The Fasting Plans are easy to navigate. Each day has a *mapped* approach. Like a map, each Fasting Plan has a starting point, a destination, and a goal.

Meditate on God's Word

Answer this question throughout the day

Pray this prayer

Note from Author: The word *unforgiveness* is not in the dictionary; however, it is a very real thing. As such, this word is used throughout this book to mean the act of not forgiving.

INTRODUCTION

Fast Answers by Beyr Reyes

What Is a Fast?

A fast is a type of sacrifice given unto the Lord, during which we make prayers, petitions, and proclamations. In other words, we choose to deny ourselves something (such as food, sweets, TV, etc.) and give it to God as an offering while we seek Him.

We fast for many reasons. We may be mourning a great loss or living in regret. At times, we feel far from God or unsure about our path. These are all good reasons, but they must not be confused with the purpose for fasting.

Fasting without purpose is futile. The purpose of the fast may be to overcome grief or depression, or to repent for something that we've done. We may fast as an attempt to get clarity for our path or to get closer to our heavenly Father. These are all purposes to fast and imply action.

The three basic elements of a fast include the purpose, the fasting agent, and the length of time. All three of these items must be clearly defined before the fast begins.

Anything placed over the worship of God is considered idolatry and flies in the face of the first two commandments. When considering your fasting agent (that thing you abstain from), the best item would be something that you find yourself putting before God: something idol-like.

Food is the traditional fasting agent—so much so that standard dictionaries define the word *fast* as abstaining from food. The Daniel Fast is the most popular food fast. (For more information, see the book *The Daniel Fast* by Susan Gregory.)

However, food is not the only (and sometimes not the best) fasting agent. We can use other things like TV, social media, caffeine, chocolate, candy, etc.—basically, things we really like.

When we deprive our body and mind of the fasting agent, it creates a longing. When we think about or crave that item, it should be a stimulus reminding us to pray and fellowship with God. This longing is a tool to remind us of how we should long for Him. The closer we draw to God, the nearer He comes to us and the louder He hears our prayers.

The key of fasting is to remember whom the fast is for and to understand that it is a time to make offerings to God. Fasting is *not* a way to show others how religious we are, and it is certainly *not* a diet.

When to Fast

Fasting, like everything else in the world, comes mainly in two forms: planned and unplanned. While often, we can see events or milestones approaching us via life's schedule, other times, we are caught off guard by unforeseen circumstances. Regardless of the situation, we can still fast effectively.

The timing for a fast comprises two considerations. You need to know *how long to fast* and *when to fast*.

So how do you know when you need to fast?

The most obvious time to fast is when God tells you to do it. He may speak to you with that small, still voice or through dreams. He may even tell you audibly or through the mouths of others. Nevertheless, when He speaks, you had better obey.

The Bible mentions several times when God instructed His children to fast corporately. Sometimes these were part of a feast and sometimes not. The proclamations generally came through kings and prophets. In today's time, this practice still exists. Churches across the world issue corporate calls to fast for various purposes.

Participation in a church corporate fast is great, but there are times when we need to fast as an individual or a family. Some reasons may include:

- For repentance
- Because you suffered a great loss
- For requests and petitions
- For deliverance
- To make a proclamation
- To seek answers and direction
- To seek God's favor or show Him honor

Sometimes you may feel a need to fast without an obvious reason. That's okay. When you don't know what to fast for, you can simply open yourself and your heart to the Holy Spirit according to Romans 8:26:

> In the same way, the Spirit helps us in our weakness. We do not know what we ought to pray for, but the Spirit himself intercedes for us through wordless groans. (NIV)

Fasting can last for one meal, one day, one week, one month, or any combination thereof. In addition, it can be a one-time thing or a recurring event. You can do a successive fast, too, like one day each week for a month.

Jesus fasted for forty days and forty nights without food. I seriously doubt very few people attempt a forty-day fast, let alone one of total abstinence from food. I personally know of only two people who tried and actually made it. When I hear their testimony, I am overtaken with awe.

More often than not, people plan their fast to be one day, one week, or twenty-one days. Another option is to fast until you note a change in the circumstances or see the fruition of your prayer. The extent of your fast should be a personal decision. Regardless of the length, define it before the fast starts and then stick to it.

Warnings About Fasting

Know the reason versus the purpose. Don't get the reason for fasting confused with the purpose for fasting. For example, take a person who is in mourning and wants to fast. The reason for the fast is the grief and pain of the mourning; the purpose of the fast is to overcome that mourning.

Plan for success. If you are planning the fast far in advance, don't set yourself up for failure. Fasting during family holidays is not advisable, and be cognizant of other special days, as well. For example, your six-year-old child will not understand why you won't eat some of her yummy birthday cake.

Keep it personal. Jesus tells us in Matthew 6:16–18 that our fasting should be seen only by God.

> *Moreover, when you fast, do not be like the hypocrites, with a sad countenance. For they disfigure their faces that they may appear to men to be fasting. Assuredly, I say to you, they have their reward. But you, when you fast, anoint your head and wash your face, so that you do not appear to men to be fasting, but to your Father who is in the secret place; and your Father who sees in secret will reward you openly.* (NKJV)

Keep it healthy. Make sure to discuss your fast beforehand with your doctor and don't fast from medicine. Don't fast from nutritious food during pregnancy. Be careful about fasting from sex with your spouse, so as to not create marital strife.

Remember whom the fast is for. Although you will be blessed for your fast, the entire act of fasting is a type of sacrifice given unto the Lord. Remember that God is asking you, "When you fasted, did you really fast for Me—for Me?" (see Zechariah 7:5).

Avoid routine. Fasting is a good thing, but like everything else, it can become routine when done too often. In the parable of the Pharisee and the tax collector, Jesus shows us an example of someone who is caught up in religious routine.

When You've Been Hurt By Others

For if you forgive men their trespasses, your heavenly Father will also forgive you. But if you do not forgive men their trespasses, neither will your Father forgive your trespasses.
　　　　　(Matthew 6:14–15 NKJV)

Fast Answers by Beyr Reyes

When You've Lost a Loved One

Job suffered more loss than anyone else in the Bible. Within one day, he lost all his livestock, servants, possessions, and children. What was Job's response? He fell to the ground and worshiped God despite the situation.

Like Job, not everyone is surrounded by a support group. He understood what it felt like to mourn considerable loss without encouragement from friends. In fact, instead of being there for him, his friends blamed him. Job called them miserable comforters.

We have help that Job didn't. We have the ultimate Comforter, the Holy Spirit, to console and reassure us in this life. In addition, we have the promise of eternal life through Jesus Christ.

Proclamation of Fast

During this fast, I avow to:
- allow myself an opportunity to grieve and welcome the Holy Spirit to comfort me.
- understand that this is only a season in my life and the enemy won't steal my peace during it.
- tell others about Jesus Christ, who died for us.

Fast Answers by Beyr Reyes

When You've Lost a Loved One
1-Day Plan

Meditate on God's Word:
For God did not appoint us to suffer wrath but to receive salvation through our Lord Jesus Christ. He died for us so that, whether we are awake or asleep, we may live together with him. Therefore encourage one another and build each other up, just as in fact you are doing. (1 Thessalonians 5:9–11 NIV)

Answer this question throughout the day:
How will I use this experience to help others who have lost loved ones?

Pray this prayer:
Dear heavenly Father, please help me to pass through this grief with the gracious help of my Comforter, the Holy Spirit. Please help me to sow these seeds of despair, pain, and confusion and to have faith in my coming season of abundant life in You. Jesus, thank You for giving Your life for me. Help me to share Your death and resurrection with others. I look for opportunities to tell others about You, Jesus, and how You helped me through this difficult time. Please help me to be an encourager for others and carry the message of Your freedom and life.

Fast Answers by Beyr Reyes

When You've Lost a Loved One
3-Day Plan

DAY 1

Meditate on God's Word:
Blessed are they that mourn: for they shall be comforted. (Jesus' words in Matthew 5:4 KJV)

Answer this question throughout the day:
Am I allowing myself to grieve and the Holy Spirit to comfort me as promised?

Pray this prayer:
Dear heavenly Father, my heart aches so deeply. If any human understands extreme grief, it would be Job. He suffered great pain, but not nearly as great as You did when You watched Your Son be tortured to death. You know the pain I feel and how to comfort me best. I graciously accept comfort from You, Holy Spirit. I remember other dark times in my life, and those, too, have passed. I believe Your Word when You say that joy is on the way. Please help me to work through this grief and put it behind me. I look forward to Your new mercies in the morning.

DAY 2

Meditate on God's Word:
To every thing there is a season, and a time to every purpose under the heaven: A time to be born, and a time to die; a time to plant, and a time to pluck up that which is planted. (Ecclesiastes 3:1–2 KJV)

Answer this question throughout the day:
What season of life am I in?

Pray this prayer:
Dear heavenly Father, I feel the lifelessness in this winter-like season of my life. In this season of death, I am reminded of the One who died for me. I reaffirm that Jesus is my Savior. He died so that I might have eternal life. Like the cold weather does for the seed of winter wheat, this cold time in my life is transforming me and I will spring forth like the hardy wheat plant in the next season. For now, I take my pain and grief and sow them as seed for my next season of growth and life. Father, I want to respond like Job did during his crises. Your Word says that, "In all this, Job did not sin by charging God with wrongdoing." Please help me to redirect my anger away from You. You are the Life-Giver, not the life-stealer. Lord, please protect me from the enemy who comes to steal, kill, and destroy.

DAY 3

Meditate on God's Word:
For God did not appoint us to suffer wrath but to receive salvation through our Lord Jesus Christ. He died for us so that, whether we are awake or asleep, we may live together with him. Therefore encourage one another and build each other up, just as in fact you are doing. (1 Thessalonians 5:9–11 NIV)

Answer this question throughout the day:
How will I use this experience to help others who have lost loved ones?

Pray this prayer:
Dear heavenly Father, please help me to pass through this grief with the gracious help of my Comforter, the Holy Spirit. Please help me to sow these seeds of despair, pain, and confusion and to have faith in my coming season of abundant life in You. Jesus, thank You for giving Your life for me. Help me to share Your death and resurrection with others. I look for opportunities to tell others about You, Jesus, and how You helped me through this difficult time. Please help me to be an encourager for others and carry the message of Your freedom and life.

Fast Answers by Beyr Reyes

When You've Lost a Loved One
7-Day Plan

DAY 1

Meditate on God's Word:
Weeping may endure for a night, but joy comes in the morning. (Psalm 30:5 NKJV)

Answer this question throughout the day:
Do I really believe that this pain and grief shall pass?

Pray this prayer:
Dear heavenly Father, my heart aches so deeply. However, I remember other dark times in my life, and those, too, have passed. I believe Your Word when You say that joy is on the way. Please help me to work through this grief and put it behind me. I look forward to Your new mercies in the morning.

DAY 2

Meditate on God's Word:
Blessed are they that mourn: for they shall be comforted. (Jesus' words in Matthew 5:4 KJV)

Answer this question throughout the day:
Am I allowing the Holy Spirit to comfort me as promised?

Pray this prayer:
Dear heavenly Father, if any human understands extreme grief, it would be Job. He suffered great pain, but not nearly as great as You did when You watched Your Son be tortured to death. You know the pain I feel and how

to comfort me best. I graciously accept comfort from You, Holy Spirit.

Day 3

Meditate on God's Word:

To every thing there is a season, and a time to every purpose under the heaven: A time to be born, and a time to die; a time to plant, and a time to pluck up that which is planted. (Ecclesiastes 3:1–2 KJV)

Answer this question throughout the day:

If I am in the cold, lifeless season of winter now, what is my next season?

Pray this prayer:

Dear heavenly Father, I feel the lifelessness in this winter-like season of my life. Like the cold weather does for the seed of winter wheat, this cold time in my life is transforming me, and I will spring forth like the hardy wheat plant in the next season. For now, I take my pain and grief and sow them as seed for my next season of growth and life.

Day 4

Meditate on God's Word:

The thief comes only to steal and kill and destroy; I have come that they may have life, and have it to the full. (John 10:10 NIV)

Answer this question throughout the day:

Is God to blame for my loss?

Pray this prayer:

Dear heavenly Father, I want to respond like Job did during his crises. Your Word says that, "In all this, Job did not sin by charging God with wrongdoing." Please help me to redirect my anger away from You. You are the Life-Giver, not the life-stealer.

DAY 5

Meditate on God's Word:
For the wages of sin is death; but the gift of God is eternal life through Jesus Christ our Lord. (Romans 6:23 KJV)

Answer this question throughout the day:
Have I accepted true, eternal life from the Life-Giver?

Pray this prayer:
Dear heavenly Father, in this season of death, I am reminded of the One who died for me. I reaffirm that Jesus is my Savior. He died so that I may have eternal life.

DAY 6

Meditate on God's Word:
But at night an angel of the Lord opened the prison doors and brought them out, and said, "Go, stand in the temple and speak to the people all the words of this life. (Acts 5:19–20 NKJV)

Answer this question throughout the day:
Am I spending more time talking about death or about the life-giving message of Jesus?

Pray this prayer:
Dear heavenly Father, despite the grief, I choose to honor You with my words instead of glorifying my pain and troubles. Thank You for freeing me from my prison cell of grief. I will tell others of Your mercy, grace, and miracles.

Day 7

Meditate on God's Word:
For God did not appoint us to suffer wrath but to receive salvation through our Lord Jesus Christ. He died for us so that, whether we are awake or asleep, we may live together with him. Therefore encourage one another and build each other up, just as in fact you are doing. (1 Thessalonians 5:9–11 NIV)

Answer this question throughout the day:
How will I use this experience to help others who have lost loved ones?

Pray this prayer:
Dear heavenly Father, please help me to pass through this grief with the gracious help of my Comforter, the Holy Spirit. Please help me to sow these seeds of despair, pain, and confusion and to have faith in my coming season of abundant life in You. Jesus, thank You for giving Your life for me. Help me to share Your death and resurrection with others. I look for opportunities to tell others about You, Jesus, and how You helped me through this difficult time. Please help me to be an encourager of others and carry the message of Your freedom and life.

Fast Answers by Beyr Reyes

When You've Been Betrayed

Jesus knew beforehand that He would be betrayed. How did He take it? The Bible says that "he was troubled in spirit." King David understood betrayal, too. What was his response? He cried out to the Lord to save him from those who persecuted him.

When people are betrayed, they have a choice. Either they turn away from the Word, allow the bitterness to create an enemy, and become a betrayer, or they forgive, move on, and pray for their betrayer. Which path will you choose?

Proclamation of Fast

During this fast, I avow to:

- overcome the hurt and forgive my betrayer.
- rebuild my trust in others and in God.
- commit to praying for my betrayer.

Fast Answers by Beyr Reyes

When You've Been Betrayed
1-Day Plan

Meditate on God's Word:
But I say to you, love your enemies, bless those who curse you, do good to those who hate you, and pray for those who spitefully use you and persecute you. (Matthew 5:44 NKJV)

Answer this question throughout the day:
Will I pray for my betrayer and for others who hurt me?

Pray this prayer:
Dear heavenly Father, this betrayal has deeply troubled my spirit. Lord, please rescue me from this pain. I put my trust in You and seek solace in Your Word. Also, please help me to forgive my betrayers as I commit myself to praying for them and others who hurt me. Lord, I choose Your way above the hurt.

Fast Answers by Beyr Reyes

When You've Been Betrayed
3-Day Plan

DAY 1

Meditate on God's Word:
For if you forgive men their trespasses, your heavenly Father will also forgive you. (Matthew 6:14 NKJV)

Answer this question throughout the day:
When will I forgive my betrayer?

Pray this prayer:
Dear heavenly Father, please help me to overcome these feelings of betrayal. Jesus, You understand betrayal better than anyone else. Please show me the proper way to handle it. Please help me with my troubled spirit. Lord, Your Word is very clear. If I forgive others, then You will forgive me. The converse is also true. If I won't forgive someone, then You won't forgive me. That is a scary thought and a situation I don't want to be in. Lord, today I choose to forgive my betrayer: not a little, not some, but completely.

DAY 2

Meditate on God's Word:
In God I have put my trust; I will not be afraid. What can man do to me? (Psalm 56:11 NKJV)

Answer this question throughout the day:
Am I afraid to trust again?

Pray this prayer:
Dear heavenly Father, right now, trust is a hard word to say, let alone something I feel like doing. I know I

can trust in You, but sometimes I have trouble. Lord, I choose today to commit my trust in You. You will never leave me nor forsake me, and I will rest in that promise. You have not given us a spirit of fear, but of power and of love and of a sound mind. I will not live in fear of being hurt again. Bitterness is a poison that will corrupt our minds and hearts. It causes us to perceive things with an ungodly attitude. Lord, my betrayer is not my enemy, and I refuse for the real enemy, satan, to make me think so. If I trust in You, who can hurt me? Yes, I could be betrayed again; however, it will *not* be my demise.

DAY 3

Meditate on God's Word:

But I say to you, love your enemies, bless those who curse you, do good to those who hate you, and pray for those who spitefully use you and persecute you. (Matthew 5:44 NKJV)

Answer this question throughout the day:

Will I pray for my betrayer and for others who hurt me?

Pray this prayer:

Dear heavenly Father, this betrayal has deeply troubled my spirit. Lord, please rescue me from this pain. I put my trust in You and seek solace in Your Word. Also, please help me to forgive my betrayers as I commit myself to praying for them and for others who hurt me. Lord, I choose Your way above the hurt.

Fast Answers by Beyr Reyes

When You've Been Betrayed
7-Day Plan

Day 1

Meditate on God's Word:
When Jesus had said these things, <u>He was troubled in spirit</u>, and testified and said, "Most assuredly, I say to you, one of you will betray Me." (John 13:21 NKJV, emphasis added)

Answer this question throughout the day:
Does Jesus understand the feelings of betrayal?

Pray this prayer:
Dear heavenly Father, please help me to overcome these feelings of betrayal. Jesus, You understand betrayal better than anyone else. Please show me the proper way to handle it. Please help me with my troubled spirit.

Day 2

Meditate on God's Word:
O LORD my God, in You I put my trust; save me from all those who persecute me; and deliver me. (Psalm 7:1 NKJV)

Answer this question throughout the day:
Do I really trust the Lord like I should?

Pray this prayer:
Dear heavenly Father, right now, trust is a hard word to say, let alone something I feel like doing. I know I

can trust in You, but sometimes I have trouble. Lord, I choose today to commit my trust in You. You will never leave me nor forsake me, and I will rest in that promise.

DAY 3

Meditate on God's Word:
For if you forgive men their trespasses, your heavenly Father will also forgive you. (Matthew 6:14 NKJV)

Answer this question throughout the day:
When will I forgive my betrayer?

Pray this prayer:
Dear heavenly Father, Your Word is very clear. If I forgive others, then you will forgive me. The converse is also true. If I won't forgive someone, then You won't forgive me. That is a scary thought and a situation I don't want to be in. Lord, today I choose to forgive my betrayer: not a little, not some, but completely.

DAY 4

Meditate on God's Word:
In God I have put my trust; I will not be afraid. What can man do to me? (Psalm 56:11 NKJV)

Answer this question throughout the day:
Am I afraid to trust my betrayer again?

Pray this prayer:
Dear heavenly Father, You have not given us a spirit of fear, but of power and of love and of a sound mind. I will not live in fear of being hurt again. If I trust in You, who can hurt me? Yes, I could be betrayed again; however, it will *not* be my demise.

Fast Answers by Beyr Reyes

Day 5

Meditate on God's Word:
At that time many will turn away from the faith and will betray and hate each other. (Matthew 24:10 NIV)

Answer this question throughout the day:
As a result of this betrayal, have I turned toward or away from the Word?

Pray this prayer:
Dear heavenly Father, I put my faith in You. Like the psalmist said, "I have restrained my feet from every evil way, that I may keep Your Word." I will run toward it and hide it in my heart. With Your Word saturating my life, I cannot develop a hate-filled heart.

Day 6

Meditate on God's Word:
Bitterly she weeps at night, tears are on her cheeks. Among all her lovers there is no one to comfort her. All her friends have betrayed her; they have become her enemies. (Lamentations 1:2 NIV)

Answer this question throughout the day:
Have I allowed the bitterness of the betrayal to create an enemy?

Pray this prayer:
Dear heavenly Father, bitterness is a poison that will corrupt our minds and hearts. It causes us to perceive things with an ungodly attitude. Lord, my betrayer is not my enemy, and I refuse for the real enemy, satan, to make me think so. Thank You, Holy Spirit, for comforting me when no one else can.

DAY 7

Meditate on God's Word:
But I say to you, love your enemies, bless those who curse you, do good to those who hate you, and pray for those who spitefully use you and persecute you. (Matthew 5:44 NKJV)

Answer this question throughout the day:
Will I pray for my betrayer and for others who hurt me?

Pray this prayer:
Dear heavenly Father, this betrayal has deeply troubled my spirit. Lord, please rescue me from this pain. I put my trust in You and seek solace in Your Word. Also, please help me to forgive my betrayers as I commit myself to praying for them and for others who hurt me. Lord, I choose Your way above the hurt.

Fast Answers by Beyr Reyes

When You've Been Cheated On

God understands the pain of adultery, so much so that He dedicated the book of Hosea to it. Hosea was married to a prostitute who wouldn't give up her ways. God uses his story to teach us how to handle adultery.

The hardest part about reading Hosea is coming to the realization that *everyone* commits adultery. Anytime we spend all our time, money, or energy on something and leave God totally out of the picture, we are cheating on Him. In the book of John, Jesus defended an adulterous woman and challenged the people to cast a stone at her only if they were without sin. The book of Hosea exemplifies God's love for us, even though we commit adultery against Him. He shows us how not to retaliate, how to forgive and to love anyway—just like He does for us.

Proclamation of Fast

During this fast, I avow to:
- get over the pain and hate.
- remove the vengeance and adultery in my own heart.
- forgive and love anyway.

Fast Answers by Beyr Reyes

When You've Been Cheated On
1-Day Plan

Meditate on God's Word:
The LORD said to me, "Go, show your love to your wife again, though she is loved by another man and is an adulteress. Love her as the LORD loves the Israelites, though they turn to other gods and love the sacred raisin cakes." (Hosea 3:1 NIV)

Answer this question throughout the day:
How should I handle this situation?

Pray this prayer:
Dear heavenly Father, You understand the pain in my heart. I know that I myself am not without the sin of adultery. So Lord, I want to forgive someone like You forgive me. No matter how much hatred I feel, I will not retaliate or seek vengeance. Instead, I choose to forgive, love anyway, and pray carefully about Your will for my next steps.

Fast Answers by Beyr Reyes

When You've Been Cheated On
3-Day Plan

DAY 1

Meditate on God's Word:
And they [the accusers of the adulterous woman] which heard it, being convicted by their own conscience, went out one by one, beginning at the eldest, even unto the last: and Jesus was left alone, and the woman standing in the midst. When Jesus had lifted up himself, and saw none but the woman, he said unto her, Woman, where are those thine accusers? hath no man condemned thee? She said, No man, Lord. And Jesus said unto her, Neither do I condemn thee: go, and sin no more. (John 8:9–11 KJV, author's addition in brackets)

Answer this question throughout the day:
If Jesus forgives adulterers, why shouldn't I?

Pray this prayer:
Dear heavenly Father, the enemy deceives us into thinking adultery is only a physical, sexual act, when in fact Your Word defines it very clearly. By Your definition, I find myself unable to count the number of times I've committed adultery in my heart. Lord, please help me to reconcile my accusations of others with those of my own. Father, You've given me an example of forgiveness by forgiving me of my adultery. How can I seriously deny someone else forgiveness for the same sin that I myself commit? Lord, please help me to offer true, heart-founded forgiveness and not just empty words. Your Word says that if someone asks for my forgiveness, I must give it over and over again. Lord, please give me the strength to forgive in my heart and actions and not just in my words.

Fast Answers by Beyr Reyes

DAY 2

Meditate on God's Word:

My heart is changed within me; all my compassion is aroused. I will not carry out my fierce anger, nor will I devastate Ephraim again. For I am God, and not a man. (Hosea 11:8–9 NIV)

Answer this question throughout the day:

Have I been retaliating and seeking vengeance?

Pray this prayer:

Dear heavenly Father, please forgive me for committing adultery against You. All those times when I could have been reading Your Word and spending time with You, I gave my attention and adoration to other things like Internet and TV. I now understand that idolatry is really adultery against You. Father, Your Word is clear about how our unfaithfulness makes You feel. In my own situation, I find myself full of hate and lacking in love. Sometimes all I want is to drive them out of my life. Lord, please teach me how to overcome this. No matter how my flesh protests, I choose not to retaliate in my anger. I know that vengeance is Yours and not mine. Lord, please help me to put away these desires to lash out and hurt the one who has hurt me. Lord, I seek to do better and treat You with the love and respect that You deserve.

DAY 3

Meditate on God's Word:

Take heed to yourselves. If your brother sins against you, rebuke him; and if he repents, forgive him. And if he sins against you seven times in a day, and seven times in a day returns to you, saying, 'I repent,' you shall forgive him. (Luke 17:3–4 NKJV)

Fast Answers by Beyr Reyes

Answer this question throughout the day:
What does it mean to truly forgive?

Pray this prayer:
Dear heavenly Father, You've given me an example of forgiveness by forgiving me of my adultery. How can I seriously deny someone else forgiveness for the same sin that I myself commit? I don't want to forgive, but I know that I must put these feelings aside and just do it. Your Word says that if someone asks for my forgiveness, I must give it over and over again. Lord, please give me the strength to forgive in my heart and actions and not just in my words. No matter how much hatred I feel, I will not retaliate or seek vengeance. Instead, I choose to forgive, to love anyway and pray carefully about Your will for my next steps.

BEEN HURT

Fast Answers by Beyr Reyes

When You've Been Cheated On
7-Day Plan

DAY 1

Meditate on God's Word:
For you have been unfaithful to your God . . . Because of all their wickedness in Gilgal, I hated them there. Because of their sinful deeds, I will drive them out of my house. I will no longer love them. (Hosea 9:1, 15 NIV)

Answer this question throughout the day:
Does God understand my pain and anguish?

Pray this prayer:
Dear heavenly Father, Your Word is clear about how our unfaithfulness makes You feel. In my own situation, I find myself full of hate and lacking in love. Sometimes all I want is to drive them out of my life. Lord, please teach me how to overcome this.

DAY 2

Meditate on God's Word:
But I tell you that anyone who looks at a woman lustfully has already committed adultery with her in his heart. (Matthew 5:28 NIV)

Answer this question throughout the day:
Have I ever committed adultery against someone else?

Pray this prayer:
Dear heavenly Father, the enemy deceives us into thinking adultery is only a physical, sexual act, when in fact Your Word defines it very clearly. By Your definition, I

find myself unable to count the number of times I've committed adultery in my heart. Lord, please help me to reconcile my accusations of others with those of my own.

DAY 3

Meditate on God's Word:
For they have committed adultery and blood is on their hands. They committed adultery with their idols; they even sacrificed their children, whom they bore to me, as food for them. (Ezekiel 23:37 NIV)

Answer this question throughout the day:
Have I ever committed adultery against God?

Pray this prayer:
Dear heavenly Father, please forgive me for committing adultery against You. All those times I could have been reading Your Word and spending time with You, I had my attention and adoration set on other things like the Internet and TV. I now understand that idolatry is really adultery against You. Thank You for this revelation. Lord, I seek to do better and treat You with the love and respect that You deserve.

DAY 4

Meditate on God's Word:
My heart is changed within me; all my compassion is aroused. I will not carry out my fierce anger, nor will I devastate Ephraim again. For I am God, and not a man. (Hosea 11:8–9 NIV)

Answer this question throughout the day:
Have I been retaliating and seeking vengeance?

Pray this prayer:
Dear heavenly Father, no matter how my flesh

protests, I choose not to retaliate in my anger. I know that vengeance is Yours and not mine. Lord, please help me to put away these desires to lash out and hurt the one who has hurt me.

DAY 5

Meditate on God's Word:

And they [the accusers of the adulterous woman] which heard it, being convicted by their own conscience, went out one by one, beginning at the eldest, even unto the last: and Jesus was left alone, and the woman standing in the midst. When Jesus had lifted up himself, and saw none but the woman, he said unto her, Woman, where are those thine accusers? Hath no man condemned thee? She said, No man, Lord. And Jesus said unto her, Neither do I condemn thee: go, and sin no more. (John 8:9–11 KJV, author's addition in brackets)

Answer this question throughout the day:

If Jesus forgives adulterers, why shouldn't I?

Pray this prayer:

Dear heavenly Father, You've given me an example of forgiveness by forgiving me of my own adultery. How can I seriously deny someone else forgiveness for the same sin that I myself commit? Lord, please help me to offer true, heart-founded forgiveness and not just empty words.

DAY 6

Meditate on God's Word:

Take heed to yourselves. If your brother sins against you, rebuke him; and if he repents, forgive him. And if he sins against you seven times in a day, and seven times in a day returns to you, saying, 'I repent,' you shall forgive him. (Luke 17:3–4 NKJV)

Fast Answers by Beyr Reyes

Answer this question throughout the day:
How many times to I need to forgive?

Pray this prayer:
Dear heavenly Father, I don't want to forgive, but I know that I must put these feelings aside and just do it. Your Word says that if someone asks for my forgiveness, I must give it over and over again. Lord, please give me the strength to forgive in my heart and actions, not just in my words.

DAY 7

Meditate on God's Word:
The LORD said to me, "Go, show your love to your wife again, though she is loved by another man and is an adulteress. Love her as the LORD loves the Israelites, though they turn to other gods and love the sacred raisin cakes." (Hosea 3:1 NIV)

Answer this question throughout the day:
What should I do after granting forgiveness?

Pray this prayer:
Dear heavenly Father, You understand the pain in my heart. I know that I myself am not without the sin of adultery. So Lord, I want to forgive someone like You forgive me. No matter how much hatred I feel, I will not retaliate or seek vengeance. Instead, I choose to forgive, to love anyway and pray carefully about Your will for my next steps.

Fast Answers by Beyr Reyes

Fast Answers by Beyr Reyes

When You've Been Stolen From

In today's society, everything seems to revolve around material things like TVs, computers, gaming systems, and the best shoes. This mindset of *having stuff* drives people to theft and coveting. Oftentimes, we justify our taking things (aka stealing) from others—things as small as office supplies from our job to items we've "borrowed" from elsewhere. The Bible tells us not to store up things as treasures because they will either be stolen or destroyed.

There is a thief in the world who is after more than our things; he's after our very life. Jesus said that the enemy comes to steal, kill, and destroy, but that He came to give abundant life. When something is stolen from us, it's not just the item that is taken. The enemy uses the circumstance to steal our joy and peace of mind.

God is the God of restoration. If we will forgive, then He will forgive us. When we pray for the thief, God begins to restore that which was stolen. His Word says that He will restore what the locusts have eaten. For Job, He restored twice as much as he had before his adversity befell him.

Proclamation of Fast

During this fast, I avow to:

- not let the true enemy steal my treasures of joy and peace of mind.
- stop justifying my own actions, especially my unforgiveness toward others.
- pray for restoration in my life and for others.

Fast Answers by Beyr Reyes

When You've Been Stolen From
1-Day Plan

Meditate on God's Word:
And the LORD restored Job's losses when he prayed for his friends. Indeed the LORD gave Job twice as much as he had before. (Job 42:10 NKJV)

Answer this question throughout the day:
When does restoration come?

Pray this prayer:
Dear heavenly Father, thank You, Lord, for Your restoring power. Job lost much more than I did, and You restored twice as much as he had. I see when it came, though. Restoration from You comes when we pray for others. Lord, I pray for the people who have stolen from me. Please meet their needs and hear their prayers. I forgive them and ask that You forgive them, too. I will seek to be an example for others who have lost things and tell them of Your forgiveness and love.

Fast Answers by Beyr Reyes

When You've Been Stolen From
3-Day Plan

DAY 1

Meditate on God's Word:
The thief cometh not, but for to steal, and to kill, and to destroy: I am come that they might have life, and that they might have it more abundantly. (John 10:10 KJV)

Answer this question throughout the day:
What treasure has the enemy stolen from me?

Pray this prayer:
Dear heavenly Father, thank You for blessing me with so much. Please help me not to let "things" fill my heart. Lord, I choose to seek treasures that are eternal instead of earthly. I understand who the real thief is, and I now realize what he has stolen—my peace of mind and joy. Like the psalmist asked, I also ask You to "restore to me the joy of Your salvation, and uphold me by Your generous Spirit." I will not let the enemy steal from me what Christ died to provide for me.

DAY 2

Meditate on God's Word:
You, therefore, who teach another, do you not teach yourself? You who preach that a man should not steal, do you steal? (Romans 2:21 NKJV)

Answer this question throughout the day:
Have I ever justified stealing or any other sin?

Fast Answers by Beyr Reyes

Pray this prayer:
Dear heavenly Father, when I consciously sin, I'm embarrassed, and many times I will make excuses for my actions. Other times, when I've stolen, I have felt entitled to the item. And then, Lord, there are times when I unknowingly steal and call it accidental. Please forgive me for trying to justify my actions, and especially my unforgiveness toward others when they do the same thing. Your Word says that if I don't forgive others, then You won't forgive me. I don't want another day to go by with the risk of You not forgiving me for my thefts because I won't forgive another. People may have stolen things from me, but I won't let them steal my right standing with You. Today is the day I will forgive them!

DAY 3

Meditate on God's Word:
And the LORD restored Job's losses when he prayed for his friends. Indeed the LORD gave Job twice as much as he had before. (Job 42:10 NKJV)

Answer this question throughout the day:
When does restoration come?

Pray this prayer:
Dear heavenly Father, thank You, Lord, for Your restoring power. Job lost much more than I did, and You restored twice as much as he had. I see when it came, though. Restoration from You comes when we pray for others. Lord, I pray for the people who have stolen from me. Please meet their needs and hear their prayers. I forgive them and ask that You forgive them, too. I will seek to be an example for others who have lost things and tell them of Your forgiveness and love.

Fast Answers by Beyr Reyes

When You've Been Stolen From
7-Day Plan

Day 1

Meditate on God's Word:
Lay not up for yourselves treasures upon earth, where moth and rust doth corrupt, and where thieves break through and steal. (Matthew 6:19 KJV)

Answer this question throughout the day:
What do I treasure?

Pray this prayer:
Dear heavenly Father, thank You for blessing me with so much. Please help me to not let "things" fill my heart. I don't want to have such an attachment to an item that it hurts me if I lose it. Lord, I choose to seek treasures that are eternal instead of earthly.

Day 2

Meditate on God's Word:
You, therefore, who teach another, do you not teach yourself? You who preach that a man should not steal, do you steal? (Romans 2:21 NKJV)

Answer this question throughout the day:
Have I ever stolen?

Pray this prayer:
Dear heavenly Father, I've stolen things—and even a few hearts. Please forgive me and help me to be a godly example for others, rather than making excuses for my behavior.

Fast Answers by Beyr Reyes

DAY 3

Meditate on God's Word:
People do not despise a thief if he steals to satisfy himself when he is starving. (Proverbs 6:30 NKJV)

Answer this question throughout the day:
Have I ever justified stealing or any other sin?

Pray this prayer:
Dear heavenly Father, when I consciously sin, I'm embarrassed, and many times I will make excuses for my actions. Other times, when I've stolen, I have felt entitled to the item. And then, Lord, there are times when I unknowingly steal and call it accidental. Please forgive me for trying to justify my actions, especially my unforgiveness toward others when they do the same thing to me.

DAY 4

Meditate on God's Word:
For if you forgive men their trespasses, your heavenly Father will also forgive you. (Matthew 6:14 NKJV)

Answer this question throughout the day:
When will I forgive those who have stolen from me?

Pray this prayer:
Dear heavenly Father, I don't want another day to go by with the risk of You not forgiving me for my thefts because I won't forgive another. People may have stolen things from me, but I won't let them steal my right standing with You. Today is the day I will forgive other people!

DAY 5

Meditate on God's Word:
So I will restore to you the years that the swarming locust has eaten. (Joel 2:25 NKJV)

Answer this question throughout the day:
Will I ever get back what was stolen?

Pray this prayer:
Dear heavenly Father, if You are able to restore as much as what a locust would eat, then how much easier will it be for You to restore the thing that was stolen from me! You are the God of restoration. Lord, it may not come back to me exactly like it was, so please give me eyes to see and ears to hear the blessings that You send. Thank You for loving me!

DAY 6

Meditate on God's Word:
The thief cometh not, but for to steal, and to kill, and to destroy: I am come that they might have life, and that they might have it more abundantly. (John 10:10 KJV)

Answer this question throughout the day:
What has the devil stolen from me?

Pray this prayer:
Dear Heavenly Father, I understand who the real thief is and I now realize what he has stolen—my peace of mind and joy. Like the psalmist asked, I also ask of You: "Restore to me the joy of Your salvation, and uphold me by Your generous Spirit." I will not let the enemy steal from me what Christ died to bless me with.

Fast Answers by Beyr Reyes

DAY 7

Meditate on God's Word:
And the LORD restored Job's losses when he prayed for his friends. Indeed the LORD gave Job twice as much as he had before. (Job 42:10 NKJV)

Answer this question throughout the day:
When does restoration come?

Pray this prayer:
Dear heavenly Father, thank You, Lord, for Your restoring power. Job lost much more than I did, and You restored twice as much as he had. I see when it came, though. Restoration from You comes when we pray for others. Lord, I pray for the people who have stolen from me. Please meet their needs and hear their prayers. I forgive them and ask that You forgive them, too. I will seek to be an example for others who have lost things and tell them of Your forgiveness and love.

Fast Answers by Beyr Reyes

When You've Been Lied About or Lied To

Jesus said that Peter would deny Him three times before the very next day. Despite Peter's bitter disagreement, he soon found himself lying three different times about being affiliated with Jesus. Later, after the resurrection, Jesus offered Peter the opportunity to restore himself.

The Bible is packed with stories about people who are full of betrayal, lies, and deceit. It teaches us ways to interact with these types and offers hope when we find ourselves in that same hot seat. The keys to success include speaking truth in love, keeping ourselves away from deceitful people, doing unto others as we would have them do unto us, and being a truthful example.

Proclamation of Fast

During this fast, I avow to:

- recognize the situation for what it is.
- remove myself from deceitful situations.
- react in a godly manner.

Fast Answers by Beyr Reyes

When You've Been Lied About or Lied To
1-Day Plan

Meditate on God's Word:
Do to others as you would have them do to you. (Luke 6:31 NIV)

Answer this question throughout the day:
What should I do to those who lie about me or to me?

Pray this prayer:
Dear heavenly Father, as I previously admitted, my flesh wants to seek revenge and set them straight. However, I must remember who the attacker is—it is the enemy, the father of lies himself. Lord, please rescue me and help me to stay out of the company of deceitful people. I choose to speak truth in love and not retaliate in hate and anger. I will treat them as I want to be treated. Lord, please help me to love them despite the circumstances and offer them an opportunity for restoration.

Fast Answers by Beyr Reyes

When You've Been Lied About or Lied To
3-Day Plan

DAY 1

Meditate on God's Word:
For the mouth of the wicked and the mouth of the deceitful have opened against me; they have spoken against me with a lying tongue. (Psalm 109:2 NKJV)

Answer this question throughout the day:
Do I really understand the situation?

Pray this prayer:
Dear heavenly Father, people are lying about me and to me. I feel like I'm under attack. I realize, though, who the attacker is. It is the enemy, the father of lies himself. I understand that he is using people to hurt me. Lord, please help me to redirect my accusations from the lying people and point them toward the true enemy. I need great discernment to see the truth. Holy Spirit, please open my eyes and ears to information that will help me to know what is truth and what is not. Help me to see the bigger picture of what is happening.

DAY 2

Meditate on God's Word:
Stretch out Your hand from above; rescue me and deliver me out of great waters, from the hand of foreigners, whose mouth speaks lying words, and whose right hand is a right hand of falsehood. (Psalm 144:7–8 NKJV)

Answer this question throughout the day:
Am I keeping myself in the line of fire?

Pray this prayer:
Dear heavenly Father, You are the great rescuer. I reach out my hand for You; please pluck me out of this mess. Please shut the mouths of the lions, like You did for Daniel in the lions' den. I admit that often I find myself influenced by the people around me. Lord, I know that staying in the company of deceitful people increases the chances of them speaking against me. Please give me the strength to break away from venomous friends. And for those family members or colleagues I can't escape, please help me remember to guard my mouth and actions when I'm with them. I want to be a truthful witness to others. Please forgive me for the times when I've lied and help me to forgive others.

DAY 3

Meditate on God's Word:
Do to others as you would have them do to you. (Luke 6:31 NIV)

Answer this question throughout the day:
What should I do to those who lie about me or to me?

Pray this prayer:
Dear heavenly Father, my flesh wants to lash out in response to the lies. Lord, I know retaliation is not Your will. You said that vengeance is Yours. I also want to jump up and defend myself, to set everything straight. However, I remember that You are my great defender. I choose to keep my fleshly intentions in check and speak truth in love instead. I won't retaliate in hate and anger. I will treat others as I want to be treated. Lord, please help me to love them despite the circumstances and to offer them an opportunity for restoration.

Fast Answers by Beyr Reyes

When You've Been Lied About or Lied To
7-Day Plan

DAY 1

Meditate on God's Word:
For the mouth of the wicked and the mouth of the deceitful have opened against me; they have spoken against me with a lying tongue. (Psalm 109:2 NKJV)

Answer this question throughout the day:
Who is speaking lies?

Pray this prayer:
Dear heavenly Father, people are lying about me and to me. I feel like I'm under attack. I realize, though, who the attacker is. It is the enemy, the father of lies himself. I understand that he is using other people to hurt me. Lord, please help me to redirect my accusations from the lying people and point them toward the true enemy. Help me to see the bigger picture of what is happening.

DAY 2

Meditate on God's Word:
And the LORD said to me, "The prophets prophesy lies in My name. I have not sent them, commanded them, nor spoken to them; they prophesy to you a false vision, divination, a worthless thing, and the deceit of their heart." (Jeremiah 14:14 NKJV)

Answer this question throughout the day:
Can I separate the truth from the lies?

Fast Answers by Beyr Reyes

Pray this prayer:
Dear heavenly Father, sometimes we are lied to by the most unexpected people, like the ones we trust. In these times, I need great discernment to see the truth. Holy Spirit, please open my eyes and ears to information that will help me to know what is truth and what is not.

Day 3

Meditate on God's Word:
Stretch out Your hand from above; rescue me and deliver me out of great waters, from the hand of foreigners, whose mouth speaks lying words, and whose right hand is a right hand of falsehood. (Psalm 144:7–8 NKJV)

Answer this question throughout the day:
Who can rescue me?

Pray this prayer:
Dear heavenly Father, You are the great rescuer. I reach out my hand for You; please pluck me out of this mess. Please shut the mouths of the lions, like You did for Daniel in the lions' den. Holy Spirit, please comfort me through the pain.

Day 4

Meditate on God's Word:
But speaking the truth in love, may grow up into him in all things, which is the head, even Christ. (Ephesians 4:15 KJV)

Answer this question throughout the day:
How do I answer the lies?

Fast Answers by Beyr Reyes

Pray this prayer:
Dear heavenly Father, my flesh wants to lash out in response to the lies. Lord, I know retaliation is not Your will. You said that vengeance is Yours. I also want to jump up and defend myself, to set everything straight. However, I remember that You are my great defender. I choose to keep my fleshly intentions in check and speak truth in love instead. I won't retaliate in hate and anger.

DAY 5

Meditate on God's Word:
He that worketh deceit shall not dwell within my house: he that telleth lies shall not tarry in my sight. (Psalm 101:7 KJV)

Answer this question throughout the day:
Am I keeping myself in the line of fire?

Pray this prayer:
Dear heavenly Father, I admit that often I find myself influenced by the people around me. Lord, I know that staying in the company of deceitful people increases the chances of them speaking against me. Please give me the strength to break away from venomous friends. And for those family members or colleagues I can't escape, please help me remember to guard my mouth and actions when I'm with them.

DAY 6

Meditate on God's Word:
A truthful witness saves lives, but a false witness is deceitful. (Proverbs 14:25 NIV)

Answer this question throughout the day:
Am I a truthful witness or do I lie, too?

Pray this prayer:
Dear heavenly Father, I want to be a truthful witness to others. Please forgive me for times when I've lied and help me to forgive others.

Day 7

Meditate on God's Word:
Do to others as you would have them do to you. (Luke 6:31 NIV)

Answer this question throughout the day:
What should I do to those who lie about me or to me?

Pray this prayer:
Dear heavenly Father, as I previously admitted, my flesh wants to seek revenge and set others straight. However, I must remember who the attacker is—it is the enemy, the father of lies himself. Lord, please rescue me and help me to stay out of the company of deceitful people. I choose to speak truth in love and not retaliate in hate and anger. I will treat them as I want to be treated. Lord, please help me to love them despite the circumstances and to offer them an opportunity for restoration.

Fast Answers by Beyr Reyes

When You've Been Forsaken

God understands what betrayal is. He experiences it daily. We betray Him with our love, we ignore His commandments, and we so easily and quickly forget what Jesus did for us on the cross.

How similar betrayal is for us, too. People betray other people the same way they do God: by renouncing their love, abandoning their covenants, forgetting the good times.

The good news is that God *never* forsakes us. No matter how wiped out we are, He is still there to pick us up. If we just remember to keep His precepts, He will make us an eternal excellence and create a joy in us that's inextinguishable by our circumstances.

Proclamation of Fast

During this fast, I avow to:

- recognize that even Jesus was forsaken.
- admit that I have forsaken others, including God.
- ensure that my situation doesn't decide my fate.

Fast Answers by Beyr Reyes

When You've Been Forsaken
1-Day Plan

Meditate on God's Word:
Whereas you have been forsaken and hated, so that no one went through you, I will make you an eternal excellence, a joy of many generations. (Isaiah 60:15 NKJV)

Answer this question throughout the day:
Will I hold on to my joy despite my circumstances?

Pray this prayer:
Dear heavenly Father, I'm sorry for the times when I have forsaken Your commandments for those when I have forgotten my first love—namely, You. Please forgive me for forsaking You and others, and thank You for *never* forsaking me. Lord, I want to follow Your precepts and love the one who forsook me even though I don't feel like it. With Your help, Holy Spirit, I will make it out of this with joy regardless of my circumstances.

Fast Answers by Beyr Reyes

When You've Been Forsaken
3-Day Plan

DAY 1

Meditate on God's Word:
And about the ninth hour Jesus cried out with a loud voice, saying, "Eli, Eli, lama sabachthani?" that is, "My God, My God, why have You forsaken Me?" (Matthew 27:46 NKJV)

Answer this question throughout the day:
Does God know how it feels to be forsaken?

Pray this prayer:
Dear heavenly Father, if anyone ever felt forsaken, it would be Jesus. We know, God, that You were not turning Your back on Jesus, but on the sin He carried to the cross for us. Jesus encountered all human emotions and feelings so that the Holy Spirit could be our ultimate Comforter. We still forsake Jesus every day, and as time moves on, each generation becomes increasingly worse. Jesus told us that we must take up our crosses and follow Him. When we do this, undoubtedly there will be times when we are forsaken by the world, too. Lord, I want to stop forsaking You and stop losing sleep over others who forsake me.

DAY 2

Meditate on God's Word:
For I, the LORD your God, am a jealous God, visiting the iniquity of the fathers upon the children to the third and fourth generations of those who hate Me, but showing mercy to thousands, to those who love Me and keep My commandments. (Exodus 20:5–6 NKJV)

Fast Answers by Beyr Reyes

Answer this question throughout the day:
Have I forsaken others, including God?

Pray this prayer:
Dear heavenly Father, I remember when I was first saved and the magnificent zeal I had. I was ready to leave everything behind just to follow You. Your first commandment says to love You with all my heart, soul, and mind. Lord, I'm sorry I have lost that love for You and Your ways. I have failed to keep the other nine commandments, as well. I have murdered others with my words, chosen things over You, stolen, and so forth. Lord, please forgive me for forsaking Your commandments and Your Word. Most of all, please forgive me for forsaking my first love—You.

Day 3

Meditate on God's Word:
Whereas you have been forsaken and hated, so that no one went through you, I will make you an eternal excellence, a joy of many generations. (Isaiah 60:15 NKJV)

Answer this question throughout the day:
Have I let my circumstances cause me to forsake God's precepts and forfeit my joy?

Pray this prayer:
Dear heavenly Father, despite the pain of my situation, I refuse to forsake Your most important precept—Jesus told us to love our neighbors as ourselves. Lord, I don't really feel like loving the one who forsook me, but I will anyway. I will not let my situation decide my fate. I'm sorry for the times when I have forsaken You and Your commandments. Please forgive me, and thank You for *never* forsaking me. With Your help, Holy Spirit, I will make it out of this with joy regardless of my circumstances.

Fast Answers by Beyr Reyes

When You've Been Forsaken
7-Day Plan

Day 1

Meditate on God's Word:
And about the ninth hour Jesus cried out with a loud voice, saying, "Eli, Eli, lama sabachthani?" that is, "My God, My God, why have You forsaken Me?" (Matthew 27:46 NKJV)

Answer this question throughout the day:
Does God know how it feels to be forsaken?

Pray this prayer:
Dear heavenly Father, if anyone ever felt forsaken, it would be Jesus. We know, God, that You were not turning Your back on Jesus, but on the sin He carried to the cross for us. Jesus encountered all human emotions and feelings so that the Holy Spirit could be our ultimate Comforter. Lord, I want to stop forsaking You. Thank You, Lord!

Day 2

Meditate on God's Word:
But first must he suffer many things, and be rejected of this generation. (Luke 17:25 KJV)

Answer this question throughout the day:
Has today's generation forsaken Jesus?

Pray this prayer:
Dear heavenly Father, I know that we forsake Jesus every day, and as time moves on, each generation

becomes increasingly worse. Jesus told us that we must take up our crosses and follow Him. When we do this, undoubtedly there will be times when we are forsaken by the world, too. Lord, I want to stop losing sleep over others who forsake me.

DAY 3

Meditate on God's Word:
Nevertheless I have this against you, that you have left your first love. (Revelation 2:4 NKJV)

Answer this question throughout the day:
Have I forsaken my first love, Jesus?

Pray this prayer:
Dear heavenly Father, I remember when I was first saved and the magnificent zeal I had. I was ready to leave everything behind just to follow You. Your first commandment says to love You with all my heart, soul, and mind. Lord, I'm sorry I have lost that love for You and Your ways. Please forgive me for forsaking my first love—You.

DAY 4

Meditate on God's Word:
For I, the LORD your God, am a jealous God, visiting the iniquity of the fathers upon the children to the third and fourth generations of those who hate Me, but showing mercy to thousands, to those who love Me and keep My commandments. (Exodus 20:5–6 NKJV)

Answer this question throughout the day:
Have I forsaken God's commandments?

Pray this prayer:
Dear heavenly Father, You know I have fallen short on

Your first commandment. However, I have failed to keep the other nine commandments, as well. I have murdered others with my words, chosen things over You, stolen, and so forth. Lord, please forgive me for forsaking Your commandments and Your Word.

DAY 5

Meditate on God's Word:
They almost wiped me from the earth, but I have not forsaken your precepts. (Psalm 119:87 NIV)

Answer this question throughout the day:
Have I let my circumstances cause me to forsake your precepts?

Pray this prayer:
Dear heavenly Father, despite the pain of my situation, I refuse to forsake Your most important precept—Jesus told us to love our neighbors as ourselves. Lord, I don't really feel like loving the one who forsook me, but I will anyway. I will not let my situation decide my fate.

DAY 6

Meditate on God's Word:
For the LORD will not reject his people; he will never forsake his inheritance. (Psalm 94:14 NIV)

Answer this question throughout the day:
Who will *never* forsake me?

Pray this prayer:
Thank You, heavenly Father, that You will *never* forsake me.

Day 7

Meditate on God's Word:
Whereas you have been forsaken and hated, so that no one went through you, I will make you an eternal excellence, a joy of many generations. (Isaiah 60:15 NKJV)

Answer this question throughout the day:
Will I hold on to my joy despite my circumstances?

Pray this prayer:
Dear heavenly Father, I'm sorry for the times when I have forsaken Your commandments and for those times when I have forgotten my first love—namely, You. Please forgive me for forsaking You and others, and thank You for *never* forsaking me. Lord, I want to follow Your precepts and love the one who forsook me, even though I don't feel like it. With Your help, Holy Spirit, I will make it out of this situation with joy regardless of my circumstances.

When You've Hurt Others

If we confess our sins, he is faithful and just to forgive us our sins, and to cleanse us from all unrighteousness.

(1 John 1:9 KJV)

Fast Answers by Beyr Reyes

When You've Betrayed Someone

When Jesus was having the Last Supper with the disciples, He announced that someone was going to betray Him. Judas immediately answered, "Lord, is it I?"

Most people envision having to answer God about their actions during the time of the Great Judgment. They fail to realize that accountability and responsibility start now.

Today is a new day and a good time for us to stop betraying God and others.

Proclamation of Fast

During this fast, I avow to:

- realize my error and accept responsibility.
- confess, repent, and ask for forgiveness.
- thank the Lord daily for forgiving me.

HURT OTHERS

Fast Answers by Beyr Reyes

When You've Betrayed Someone
1-Day Plan

Meditate on God's Word:
Blessed is he whose transgression is forgiven, whose sin is covered. (Psalm 32:1 KJV)

Answer this question throughout the day:
Have I thanked God for my forgiveness through Jesus Christ?

Pray this prayer:
Dear heavenly Father, I regret my betrayal of You and others and I take responsibility for each time. I confess my sin to You and them, and seek true repentance by stopping the betrayal and starting to do what is right. Thank You for forgiving me. Thank You, Jesus, for carrying my sins to the cross and dying for me.

Fast Answers by Beyr Reyes

When You've Betrayed Someone
3-Day Plan

DAY 1

Meditate on God's Word:
Then Judas, who was betraying Him, answered and said, "Rabbi, is it I?" He said to him, "You have said it." (Matthew 26:25 NKJV)

Answer this question throughout the day:
Have I accepted responsibility for my act of betrayal?

Pray this prayer:
Dear heavenly Father, one of the hardest things to do is to own up to sin. I realize my error and accept responsibility for my actions. Please forgive me for the times when I'm not loyal to You and Your Word, as well. Lord, please forgive me for being sorry for the wrong reasons. I want to be sorry that I sinned and not sorry because I'm worried that others will think bad of me. Only godly sorrow leads to true repentance.

DAY 2

Meditate on God's Word:
Confess your trespasses to one another, and pray for one another, that you may be healed. The effective, fervent prayer of a righteous man avails much. (James 5:16 NKJV)

Answer this question throughout the day:
Have I confessed my betrayal and asked for forgiveness?

Fast Answers by Beyr Reyes

Pray this prayer:
Dear heavenly Father, Your Word says that before I come to You with offerings, I must first reconcile with my brother; therefore, I will waste no more time in confessing my actions to the person I betrayed and asking for their forgiveness. I will not make excuses for what I've done. I understand that repenting is not the same as being sorry. Repentance means that I stop the action and start doing what is right. Today, I chose to repent from betraying people. Lord, please forgive me for betraying You and others. Holy Spirit, please quicken my heart concerning other times when I've committed betrayal so that I can address them, too.

DAY 3

Meditate on God's Word:
Blessed is he whose transgression is forgiven, whose sin is covered. (Psalm 32:1 KJV)

Answer this question throughout the day:
Have I thanked God for my forgiveness through Jesus Christ?

Pray this prayer:
Dear heavenly Father, I regret my betrayal of You and others and take responsibility for each time. I confess my sin to you and them, and I seek true repentance by stopping the betrayals and starting to do what is right. Thank You for forgiving me. Thank You, Jesus, for carrying my sins to the cross and dying for me.

Fast Answers by Beyr Reyes

When You've Betrayed Someone
7-Day Plan

DAY 1

Meditate on God's Word:
Then Judas, who was betraying Him, answered and said, "Rabbi, is it I?" He said to him, "You have said it." (Matthew 26:25 NKJV)

Answer this question throughout the day:
Have I accepted responsibility for my act of betrayal?

Pray this prayer:
Dear heavenly Father, one of the hardest things to do is to own up to sin. I realize my error and accept responsibility for my actions. Lord, please help me to be strong and not back down.

DAY 2

Meditate on God's Word:
For godly sorrow produces repentance leading to salvation, not to be regretted; but the sorrow of the world produces death. (2 Corinthians 7:10 NKJV)

Answer this question throughout the day:
Am I experiencing worldly sorrow or godly sorrow?

Pray this prayer:
Dear heavenly Father, I feel sorrowful for my actions. But, Lord, please forgive me for being sorry for the wrong reasons. I want to be sorry that I sinned and not because I'm worried that others will think bad of me. Only godly sorrow leads to true repentance.

Day 3

Meditate on God's Word:
Confess your trespasses to one another, and pray for one another, that you may be healed. The effective, fervent prayer of a righteous man avails much. (James 5:16 NKJV)

Answer this question throughout the day:
Have I confessed my actions to the person I betrayed and to God?

Pray this prayer:
Dear heavenly Father, Your Word says that before I come to You with offerings, I must first reconcile with my brother; therefore, I will waste no more time in confessing my actions to the person I betrayed and asking for their forgiveness. I will not make excuses for what I've done.

Day 4

Meditate on God's Word:
The Son of Man will go just as it is written about him. But woe to that man who betrays the Son of Man! It would be better for him if he had not been born. (Mark 14:21 NIV)

Answer this question throughout the day:
Have I ever betrayed God?

Pray this prayer:
Dear heavenly Father, the ultimate betrayal is when we betray You. Please forgive me for the times when I'm not loyal to You and Your Word.

DAY 5

Meditate on God's Word:
Now I rejoice, not that you were made sorry, but that your sorrow led to repentance. (2 Corinthians 7:9 NKJV)

Answer this question throughout the day:
When will I repent of my hurtful actions?

Pray this prayer:
Dear heavenly Father, I understand that repenting is not the same as being sorry. Repentance means that I stop the action and start doing what is right. Today, I choose to repent from betraying people.

DAY 6

Meditate on God's Word:
For the sake of your name, Lord, forgive my iniquity, though it is great. (Psalm 25:11 NIV)

Answer this question throughout the day:
Have I asked God for forgiveness?

Pray this prayer:
Dear heavenly Father, please forgive me for betraying You and others. Holy Spirit, please quicken my heart concerning other times when I've committed betrayal so that I can address them, too.

DAY 7

Meditate on God's Word:
Blessed is he whose transgression is forgiven, whose sin is covered. (Psalm 32:1 KJV)

Fast Answers by Beyr Reyes

A**nswer this question throughout the day:**
Have I thanked God for my forgiveness through Jesus Christ?

P**ray this prayer:**
Dear heavenly Father, I regret my betrayal of You and others, and I take responsibility for each time. I confess my sin to You and them, and seek true repentance by stopping the betrayals and starting to do what is right. Thank You for forgiving me. Thank You, Jesus, for carrying my sins to the cross and dying for me.

Fast Answers by Beyr Reyes

When You've Committed Adultery

In Matthew, the Bible says that anyone who looks at another person with lustful intent has already committed adultery in his or her heart. In the book of John, Jesus defended an adulterous woman and challenged to people to cast a stone at her only if they were without sin. Basically—everyone is an adulterer. (But that's not a license to do it.)

The hardest part about reading the book of Hosea is coming to the realization that *everyone* commits adultery against God. Anytime we spend all our time, money, or energy on something else and leave God totally out of the picture, we are cheating on Him. The book of Hosea exemplifies God's love for us, even though we commit adultery against Him all the time.

The key to dealing with adultery is to seek forgiveness, repent of your actions, and then find ways to curtail future temptations.

Proclamation of Fast

During this fast, I avow to:

- realize my error and accept responsibility.
- confess, repent, and ask for forgiveness.
- find ways to remove myself from temptation.

Fast Answers by Beyr Reyes

When You've Committed Adultery
1-Day Plan

Meditate on God's Word:
For if anyone is a hearer of the word and not a doer, he is like a man observing his natural face in a mirror; for he observes himself, goes away, and immediately forgets what kind of man he was. But he who looks into the perfect law of liberty and continues in it, and is not a forgetful hearer but a doer of the work, this one will be blessed in what he does. (James 1:23–25 NKJV)

Answer this question throughout the day:
Have I really changed, or am I just talking my way out of my sin?

Pray this prayer:
Dear heavenly Father, I confess my sin to You and my loved one. I ask You for forgiveness. Lord, I don't want to be an adulterous person. I repent of this sin and ask that You open my eyes to future temptations. Help me to find ways to remove myself from tempting situations. When I remember this event, I will praise Your name and tell others of Your mercies. I will show them a changed person.

Fast Answers by Beyr Reyes

When You've Committed Adultery
3-Day Plan

DAY 1

Meditate on God's Word:
They said to Him, "Teacher, this woman was caught in adultery, in the very act." (John 8:4 NKJV)

Answer this question throughout the day:
Have I really acknowledged my error, or am I just acting because I was caught?

Pray this prayer:
Dear heavenly Father, I don't want to add fraud to my list of errors. I admit that I am remorseful for getting caught. However, I am more sorry for committing the act of adultery in the first place. Please help me to put aside my fleshly inclinations and truly acknowledge my sin. I understand that we, as the Church, are the Bride of Christ, Your anointed ones. Many times I have fallen away from You and sought answers from high places. I'm sorry, Lord, for cheating on You and others. Please forgive me.

DAY 2

Meditate on God's Word:
He who covers his sins will not prosper, But whoever confesses and forsakes them will have mercy. (Proverbs 28:13 NKJV)

Answer this question throughout the day:
When will I confess my adultery to my loved one, ask for forgiveness, and repent?

Pray this prayer:
Dear heavenly Father, I will not procrastinate anymore. I will confess my adultery to my loved one. I will ask them to forgive me for the adultery, as well as for the pain I've caused. Lord, please give me the strength and the right words to say. Adultery is a wicked sin that I've committed against You and others. I repent from these actions and ask that You help me to remove the desires from my mind. I will not turn back ever again.

DAY 3

Meditate on God's Word:
For if anyone is a hearer of the word and not a doer, he is like a man observing his natural face in a mirror; for he observes himself, goes away, and immediately forgets what kind of man he was. But he who looks into the perfect law of liberty and continues in it, and is not a forgetful hearer but a doer of the work, this one will be blessed in what he does. (James 1:23–25 NKJV)

Answer this question throughout the day:
Have I really changed, or am I just talking my way out of my sin?

Pray this prayer:
Dear heavenly Father, I confess my sin to You and my loved one. I ask You for forgiveness. Lord, I don't want to be an adulterous person. I repent of this sin and ask that You open my eyes to future temptations. Help me to find ways to remove myself from tempting situations. When I remember this event, I will praise Your name and tell others of Your mercies. I will show them that I am a changed person.

Fast Answers by Beyr Reyes

When You've Committed Adultery
7-Day Plan

DAY 1

Meditate on God's Word:
They said to Him, "Teacher, this woman was caught in adultery, in the very act." (John 8:4 NKJV)

Answer this question throughout the day:
Have I really acknowledged my error, or am I just acting because I was caught?

Pray this prayer:
Dear heavenly Father, I don't want to add fraud to my list of errors. I admit that I am remorseful for getting caught. However, I am more sorry for committing the act of adultery in the first place. Please help me to put aside my fleshly inclinations and truly acknowledge my sin.

DAY 2

Meditate on God's Word:
He who covers his sins will not prosper, but whoever confesses and forsakes them will have mercy. (Proverbs 28:13 NKJV)

Answer this question throughout the day:
When will I confess my adultery to my loved one?

Pray this prayer:
Dear heavenly Father, I will not procrastinate anymore. I will confess my adultery to my loved one and ask for forgiveness. Lord, please give me the strength and the right words to say.

HURT OTHERS

Fast Answers by Beyr Reyes

Day 3

Meditate on God's Word:
During the reign of King Josiah, the LORD said to me, "Have you seen what faithless Israel [God's anointed people] *has done? She has gone up on every high hill and under every spreading tree and has committed adultery there."* (Jeremiah 3:6 NIV, author's addition in brackets)

Answer this question throughout the day:
Have I ever cheated on God?

Pray this prayer:
Dear heavenly Father, I understand that we, as the Church, are the Bride of Christ, Your anointed ones. Many times I have fallen away from You and sought answers from high places. I'm sorry, Lord, for cheating on You. Please forgive me.

Day 4

Meditate on God's Word:
Repent of this wickedness and pray to the Lord in the hope that he may forgive you for having such a thought in your heart. (Acts 8:22 NIV)

Answer this question throughout the day:
When will I repent of my adulterous sin?

Pray this prayer:
Dear heavenly Father, adultery is a wicked sin that I've committed against You and others. I repent from these actions and ask that You help remove the desires from my mind. I will not turn back ever again.

Fast Answers by Beyr Reyes

Day 5

Meditate on God's Word:
Look upon mine affliction and my pain; and forgive all my sins. (Psalm 25:18 KJV)

Answer this question throughout the day:
Have I asked forgiveness from my loved one?

Pray this prayer:
Dear heavenly Father, I will wait no longer to ask my loved one for forgiveness. I will ask them to forgive me for the adultery, as well as for the pain I've caused. Lord, please help me to speak with love.

Day 6

Meditate on God's Word:
No temptation has overtaken you except what is common to mankind. And God is faithful; he will not let you be tempted beyond what you can bear. But when you are tempted, he will also provide a way out so that you can endure it. (1 Corinthians 10:13 NIV)

Answer this question throughout the day:
What actions will I take to ensure this will never happen again?

Pray this prayer:
Dear heavenly Father, when I am tempted to commit adultery again, thank You for providing a way out. Holy Spirit, please open my eyes to see my escape, and help me to withstand and endure future temptation.

DAY 7

Meditate on God's Word:
For if anyone is a hearer of the word and not a doer, he is like a man observing his natural face in a mirror; for he observes himself, goes away, and immediately forgets what kind of man he was. But he who looks into the perfect law of liberty and continues in it, and is not a forgetful hearer but a doer of the work, this one will be blessed in what he does. (James 1:23–25 NKJV)

Answer this question throughout the day:
Have I really changed, or am I just talking my way out of my sin?

Pray this prayer:
Dear heavenly Father, I confess my sin to You and my loved one. I ask You for forgiveness. Lord, I don't want to be an adulterous person. I repent of this sin and ask that You open my eyes to future temptations. Help me to find ways to remove myself from tempting situations. When I remember this event, I will praise Your name and tell others of Your mercies. I will show them I am a changed person.

Fast Answers by Beyr Reyes

When You Need Forgiveness

We all need forgiveness for something or another. But before we can be forgiven, we must first seek it—both from the one we've sinned against and from God.

In Matthew, we are told that if when making an offering to God we remember that someone has something against us, we must leave our gift at the altar, go reconcile the relationship, and then come back and finish the offering.

God's forgiveness is only through the blood of Jesus. Once we accept Jesus as our Lord and Savior, He removes our transgressions as far from us as the east is from the west. How far? you might ask. As someone so aptly put it: from one nailed hand to the other.

Proclamation of Fast

During this fast, I avow to:

- seek forgiveness from the ones I sinned against and from God.
- believe that I'm really forgiven.
- tell others of my forgiveness through Jesus.

Fast Answers by Beyr Reyes

When You Need Forgiveness
1-Day Plan

Meditate on God's Word:
Only take heed to yourself, and diligently keep yourself, lest you forget the things your eyes have seen, and lest they depart from your heart all the days of your life. And teach them to your children and your grandchildren. (Deuteronomy 4:9 NKJV)

Answer this question throughout the day:
Will I tell others of God's forgiveness?

Pray this prayer:
Dear heavenly Father, I choose to call upon Your name, confess my sins, and repent of my ways. I understand that true forgiveness is only found through Jesus. Your Word says that if we forgive people their trespasses, then You will also forgive us. Lord, if there is anyone I haven't forgiven, please bring their name to my mind. Thank You for Your forgiveness. I will remember my experience and tell others of Your mercy and forgiveness all the days of my life.

Fast Answers by Beyr Reyes

When You Need Forgiveness
3-Day Plan

Day 1

Meditate on God's Word:
If My people who are called by My name will humble themselves, and pray and seek My face, and turn from their wicked ways, then I will hear from heaven, and will forgive their sin and heal their land. (2 Chronicles 7:14 NKJV)

Answer this question throughout the day:
How do I seek forgiveness from the Lord?

Pray this prayer:
Dear heavenly Father, I humbly call upon Your name to forgive me. I will depart from my sinful ways and will seek only You and Your kingdom. I confess my sins to You. Please cleanse me from all unrighteousness.

Day 2

Meditate on God's Word:
Therefore, my friends, I want you to know that through Jesus the forgiveness of sins is proclaimed to you. (Acts 13:38 NIV)

Answer this question throughout the day:
Am I *really* forgiven?

Pray this prayer:
Dear heavenly Father, I know that ultimate forgiveness comes only through Jesus. Thank You, Jesus, for dying for me. Lord, Your Word says that we must forgive or we won't be forgiven. Today, I chose to forgive everyone who

has ever hurt me. I especially forgive myself. Holy Spirit, please help me to have faith that I'm forgiven. It's one thing to be told that we are, but it's another to believe it. Lord, I thank You and accept Your forgiveness in my life.

DAY 3

Meditate on God's Word:
Only take heed to yourself, and diligently keep yourself, lest you forget the things your eyes have seen, and lest they depart from your heart all the days of your life. And teach them to your children and your grandchildren. (Deuteronomy 4:9 NKJV)

Answer this question throughout the day:
Will I tell others of God's forgiveness?

Pray this prayer:
Dear heavenly Father, I choose to call upon Your name, confess my sins, and repent of my ways. I understand that true forgiveness is only found through Jesus. Your Word says that if we forgive people their trespasses, then You will also forgive us. Lord, if there is anyone I haven't forgiven, please bring their name to my mind. Thank You for Your forgiveness. I will remember my experience and tell others of Your mercy and forgiveness all the days of my life.

Fast Answers by Beyr Reyes

When You Need Forgiveness
7-Day Plan

Day 1

Meditate on God's Word:
If My people who are called by My name will humble themselves, and pray and seek My face, and turn from their wicked ways, then I will hear from heaven, and will forgive their sin and heal their land. (2 Chronicles 7:14 NKJV)

Answer this question throughout the day:
Whom should I call upon?

Pray this prayer:
Dear heavenly Father, I humbly call upon Your name to forgive me. I will depart from my sinful ways and will seek only You and Your kingdom.

Day 2

Meditate on God's Word:
If we confess our sins, he is faithful and just to forgive us our sins, and to cleanse us from all unrighteousness. (1 John 1:9 KJV)

Answer this question throughout the day:
What should I confess?

Pray this prayer:
Dear heavenly Father, I confess my sins to You. I want to be cleansed from all unrighteousness. [Name sins and confess them.]

Fast Answers by Beyr Reyes

DAY 3

Meditate on God's Word:
Therefore, my friends, I want you to know that through Jesus the forgiveness of sins is proclaimed to you. (Acts 13:38 NIV)

Answer this question throughout the day:
In whose name is true forgiveness found?

Pray this prayer:
Dear heavenly Father, I know that ultimate forgiveness only comes through Jesus. Lord, I thank You and accept Your forgiveness in my life.

DAY 4

Meditate on God's Word:
Repent therefore of this thy wickedness, and pray God, if perhaps the thought of thine heart may be forgiven thee. (Acts 8:22 KJV)

Answer this question throughout the day:
Do I understand what "repent" means?

Pray this prayer:
Dear heavenly Father, I understand that repenting is not the same as being sorry. Repentance means that I stop the action and start doing what is right. Today, I chose to repent from my sins.

DAY 5

Meditate on God's Word:
But if you do not forgive men their trespasses, neither will your Father forgive your trespasses. (Matthew 6:15 NKJV)

Fast Answers by Beyr Reyes

Answer this question throughout the day:
Is there anyone I haven't forgiven?

Pray this prayer:
Dear heavenly Father, many people have hurt me in the past, and I've held on to unforgiveness. Lord, Your Word says that we must forgive or we won't be forgiven. Today, I choose to forgive everyone who has ever hurt me. I especially forgive myself.

DAY 6

Meditate on God's Word:
And the prayer offered in faith will make the sick person well; the Lord will raise them up. If they have sinned, they will be forgiven. (James 5:15 NIV)

Answer this question throughout the day:
Am I *really* forgiven?

Pray this prayer:
Dear heavenly Father, please help me to have faith that I'm forgiven. It's one thing to be told that I am, but it's another to believe it. If Your Word says it's so, then it is.

DAY 7

Meditate on God's Word:
Only take heed to yourself, and diligently keep yourself, lest you forget the things your eyes have seen, and lest they depart from your heart all the days of your life. And teach them to your children and your grandchildren. (Deuteronomy 4:9 NKJV)

Answer this question throughout the day:
Will I tell others of God's forgiveness?

Pray this prayer:
Dear heavenly Father, I choose to call upon Your name, confess my sins, and repent of my ways. I understand that true forgiveness is only found through Jesus. Your Word says that if we forgive people their trespasses, then You will also forgive us. Lord, if there is anyone I haven't forgiven, please bring their name to my mind. Thank You for Your forgiveness. I will remember my experience and tell others of Your mercy and forgiveness all the days of my life.

Fast Answers by Beyr Reyes

When You've Stolen from Someone

Everything belongs to the Lord. *Everything.* Any time we steal from people, we are stealing also from God.

Thieves fail to realize that every day someone else is stealing something very important from them. Our enemy, the devil, steals right-mindedness and convinces people to justify their thefts. He tricks them into a sinful, self-indulgent existence and causes them to forfeit their very lives.

According to Jeremiah 2:26, a thief is ashamed when he is caught. However, the big question is: is the shame derived from the regret over sinning or from the worries about what others may think of him when they find out? There is a difference between godly sorrow and worldly sorrow, and only godly sorrow leads to true repentance.

Proclamation of Fast

During this fast, I avow to:

- realize that everything is the Lord's and that when I steal, I'm stealing from Him, too.
- stop stealing, stop justifying, and make recompense.
- repent and take back right-mindedness.

Fast Answers by Beyr Reyes

When You've Stolen from Someone
1-Day Plan

Meditate on God's Word:
The thief cometh not, but for to steal, and to kill, and to destroy: I am come that they might have life, and that they might have it more abundantly. (John 10:10 KJV)

Answer this question throughout the day:
What has really been stolen?

Pray this prayer:
Dear heavenly Father, the enemy stole my thoughts and encouraged me to think it was okay to steal. Please help me to take back my right-mindedness. I repent of my actions. Everything is Yours, and I refuse to steal from You any longer. I will stop justifying my actions and give back what I've taken. Lord, I will not waste time.

Fast Answers by Beyr Reyes

When You've Stolen from Someone
3-Day Plan

Day 1

Meditate on God's Word:
"Will a man rob God? Yet you have robbed Me! But you say, 'In what way have we robbed You?' In tithes and offerings. You are cursed with a curse, For you have robbed Me, Even this whole nation. Bring all the tithes into the storehouse, That there may be food in My house, And try Me now in this," Says the LORD of hosts, "If I will not open for you the windows of heaven And pour out for you such blessing That there will not be room enough to receive it. (Malachi 3:8–10 NKJV)

Answer this question throughout the day:
What am I stealing from God?

Pray this prayer:
Dear heavenly Father, everything belongs to You. When I steal, not only am I stealing from an individual, but I'm also stealing from You. Lord, please help me to change my mindset about material items and to realize true ownership and the consequences of theft. Please forgive me for the times when I thought tithing was just something preachers made up to get money. Please open my mind to the idea that tithing isn't just about money. It also deals with our time and other nonmonetary blessings. I will no longer rob God of what He commands and desires.

Day 2

Meditate on God's Word:
If they give back what they took in pledge for a loan, return what they have stolen, follow the decrees that

give life, and do no evil—that person will surely live; they will not die. (Ezekiel 33:15 NIV)

Answer this question throughout the day:
When will I stop stealing, stop justifying my sin, and make recompense?

Pray this prayer:
Dear heavenly Father, when I consciously sin, I'm embarrassed and many times will make excuses for my actions. Other times when I've stolen, I have felt entitled to the item. And then, Lord, there are times when I unknowingly steal and call it accidental. Please forgive me for trying to justify my actions. Today is the day when I will stop stealing. No longer will I take things that are not mine. Instead, I will use my hands to share with those in need and to return all that I have stolen.

DAY 3

Meditate on God's Word:
The thief cometh not, but for to steal, and to kill, and to destroy: I am come that they might have life, and that they might have it more abundantly. (John 10:10 KJV)

Answer this question throughout the day:
What has the enemy stolen from me?

Pray this prayer:
Dear heavenly Father, the enemy stole my thoughts and encouraged me to think it was okay to steal. Please help me to take back my right-mindedness. I repent of my actions. Everything is Yours, and I refuse to steal from You any longer. I will stop justifying my actions and give back what I've taken. Lord, I will not waste time.

Fast Answers by Beyr Reyes

When You've Stolen from Someone
7-Day Plan

Day 1

Meditate on God's Word:
The earth is the Lord's, and everything in it, the world, and all who live in it. (Psalm 24:1 NIV)

Answer this question throughout the day:
Who owns everything?

Pray this prayer:
Dear heavenly Father, everything belongs to You. When I steal, not only am I stealing from an individual, but I'm also stealing from You. Lord, please help me to change my mindset about material items and to realize true ownership and the consequences of theft.

Day 2

Meditate on God's Word:
"Will a man rob God? Yet you have robbed Me! But you say, 'In what way have we robbed You?' In tithes and offerings. You are cursed with a curse, For you have robbed Me, Even this whole nation. Bring all the tithes into the storehouse, That there may be food in My house, And try Me now in this," Says the Lord of hosts, "If I will not open for you the windows of heaven And pour out for you such blessing That there will not be room enough to receive it. (Malachi 3:8–10 NKJV)

Answer this question throughout the day:
What am I stealing from God?

Pray this prayer:
Dear heavenly Father, please forgive me for the times when I thought tithing was just something preachers made up to get money. Please open my mind to the idea that tithing isn't just about money. It also deals with our time and other nonmonetary blessings. I will no longer rob God of what He commands and desires.

Day 3

Meditate on God's Word:
Men do not despise a thief, if he steal to satisfy his soul when he is hungry. (Proverbs 6:30 KJV)

Answer this question throughout the day:
Am I justifying this or any other sin?

Pray this prayer:
Dear heavenly Father, when I consciously sin, I'm embarrassed and many times will make excuses for my actions. Other times when I've stolen, I have felt entitled to the item. And then, Lord, there are times when I unknowingly steal and call it accidental. Please forgive me for trying to justify my actions.

Day 4

Meditate on God's Word:
Anyone who has been stealing must steal no longer, but must work, doing something useful with their own hands, that they may have something to share with those in need. (Ephesians 4:28 NIV)

Answer this question throughout the day:
Will I stop stealing?

Pray this prayer:
Dear heavenly Father, today is the day when I will stop stealing. No longer will I take things that are not mine. Instead, I will use my hands to share with those in need.

DAY 5

Meditate on God's Word:
If they give back what they took in pledge for a loan, return what they have stolen, follow the decrees that give life, and do no evil—that person will surely live; they will not die. (Ezekiel 33:15 NIV)

Answer this question throughout the day:
Have I returned what I've stolen?

Pray this prayer:
Dear heavenly Father, I will return all that I have stolen. In situations where I no longer have the item, I will make a generous recompense in another way.

DAY 6

Meditate on God's Word:
For yourselves know perfectly that the day of the Lord so cometh as a thief in the night. (1 Thessalonians 5:2 KJV)

Answer this question throughout the day:
Am I dragging my feet to do what God asks me to do?

Pray this prayer:
Dear heavenly Father, I will not procrastinate anymore. I shudder to think that you would return before I make amends. I will be quick and not waste time.

Day 7

Meditate on God's Word:
The thief cometh not, but for to steal, and to kill, and to destroy: I am come that they might have life, and that they might have it more abundantly. (John 10:10 KJV)

Answer this question throughout the day:
What has the enemy stolen from me?

Pray this prayer:
Dear heavenly Father, the enemy stole my thoughts and encouraged me to think it was okay to steal. Please help me to take back my right-mindedness. I repent of my actions. Everything is Yours, and I refuse to steal from You any longer. I will stop justifying my actions and give back what I've taken. Lord, I will not waste time.

Fast Answers by Beyr Reyes

When You've Lied

The Bible is packed with stories about people who are full of betrayal, lies, and deceit. It also gives grave warnings for people who continue in these ways.

The enemy, also known as the father of lies, uses deceit as his main weapon. He twists our thinking and causes us to operate in sin. For example, in the book of Acts, when all the early believers agreed to share all their possessions, one husband and wife decided that it would be okay to hold a little back. How were they received in the offering line? Peter asked them, "Ananias, how is it that Satan has so filled your heart that you have lied to the Holy Spirit and have kept for yourself some of the money you received for the land? ... What made you think of doing such a thing? You have not lied just to human beings but to God" (Acts 5:3–4 NIV). After Ananias heard this, he fell dead. When they brought the wife in, she lied, too, and fell dead. How many times in our lives have we thought that a little white lie wouldn't hurt?

Jesus understood the power of truth and deception and even made a special prayer request for His disciples, "Sanctify them by the truth. Your word is truth" (John 17:17 NIV). He later told them that "you will know the truth, and the truth will make you free" (John 8:32 NIV).

Proclamation of Fast

During this fast, I avow to:

- walk blamelessly, speak righteously, and live freely.
- address the root of my lying problem and retrain my mouth.
- use every opportunity to rightly handle the truth.

Fast Answers by Beyr Reyes

When You've Lied
1-Day Plan

Meditate on God's Word:
Be diligent to present yourself approved to God, a worker who does not need to be ashamed, rightly dividing the word of truth. (2 Timothy 2:15 NKJV)

Answer this question throughout the day:
Will I commit to start rightly handling truth?

Pray this prayer:
Dear heavenly Father, I want to be set free from the spirit of lying. Please help me to identify the root of my lying problem. I want to present myself approved to You. Holy Spirit, please lead me in Your truthful ways and help me to retrain my mouth. When I am reminded of the times I lied, I put Your Word on my lips and speak only what is righteous. Living a life of truth will set me free, so today I will start rightly handling truth.

Fast Answers by Beyr Reyes

When You've Lied
3-Day Plan

Day 1

Meditate on God's Word:
Jesus said, *"If you hold to my teaching, you are really my disciples. Then you will know the truth, and the truth will set you free."* (John 8:31–32 NIV)

Answer this question throughout the day:
What will truth do for me?

Pray this prayer:
Dear heavenly Father, I want to be the type of person You keep close to You. Holy Spirit, please help me to speak truth from my heart, to utter no slander nor slur against another, and to walk blamelessly. I chose to speak only what is righteous. Lies are like chains that bind me. I want to be free. I understand now that living a life of truth will set me free.

Day 2

Meditate on God's Word:
Everyone will deceive his neighbor, and will not speak the truth; they have taught their tongue to speak lies; they weary themselves to commit iniquity. (Jeremiah 9:5 NKJV)

Answer this question throughout the day:
Do I know the root of my lying problem and realize who taught me to speak lies?

Pray this prayer:
Dear heavenly Father, oh, how I want to blame others for teaching me to lie, but in reality I know that I taught myself. I'm not fooling anyone. There is a reason that I lie. Many times the lie is born out of an emotion such as fear. Holy Spirit, please help me to retrain my mouth and to identify and deal with the root of my lying problem. Like the psalmist said, "I will keep my tongue from evil and my lips from telling lies." Instead of lying, my tongue will proclaim Your righteousness and Your praises all day long. Holy Spirit, please come alongside of me and help me to guard my mouth. Lead me in Your truth and teach me Your truthful ways.

DAY 3

Meditate on God's Word:
Be diligent to present yourself approved to God, a worker who does not need to be ashamed, rightly dividing the word of truth. (2 Timothy 2:15 NKJV)

Answer this question throughout the day:
Will I commit to start rightly handling truth?

Pray this prayer:
Dear heavenly Father, I want to be set free from the spirit of lying. Please help me to identify the root of my lying problem. I want to present myself approved to You. Holy Spirit, please lead me in Your truthful ways and help me to retrain my mouth. When I am reminded of the times I lied, I put Your Word on my lips and speak only what is righteous. Living a life of truth will set me free, so today I will start rightly handling truth.

Fast Answers by Beyr Reyes
When You've Lied
7-Day Plan

Day 1

Meditate on God's Word:
LORD, who may dwell in your sacred tent? Who may live on your holy mountain? The one whose walk is blameless, who does what is righteous, who speaks the truth from their heart; whose tongue utters no slander, who does no wrong to a neighbor, and casts no slur on others. (Psalm 15:1–3 NIV)

Answer this question throughout the day:
What kind of person does the Lord keep close?

Pray this prayer:
Dear heavenly Father, I want to be the type of person You keep close to You. Holy Spirit, please help me to speak truth from my heart and to utter no slander nor slur against another. I chose to speak only what is righteous.

Day 2

Meditate on God's Word:
Jesus said, "If you hold to my teaching, you are really my disciples. Then you will know the truth, and the truth will set you free." (John 8:31–32 NIV)

Answer this question throughout the day:
What will truth do for me?

Pray this prayer:
Dear heavenly Father, lies are like chains that bind me. I want to be free. I understand now that living a

life of truth will set me free.

Day 3

Meditate on God's Word:
Everyone will deceive his neighbor, and will not speak the truth; they have taught their tongue to speak lies; they weary themselves to commit iniquity. (Jeremiah 9:5 NKJV)

Answer this question throughout the day:
Have I taught myself to speak lies?

Pray this prayer:
Dear heavenly Father, oh, how I want to blame others for teaching me to lie, but in reality I know that I taught myself. Lord, I need to retrain my mouth. Like the psalmist said, "I will keep my tongue from evil and my lips from telling lies." Instead of lying, my tongue will proclaim Your righteousness and Your praises all day long.

Day 4

Meditate on God's Word:
Lead me in thy truth, and teach me: for thou art the God of my salvation; on thee do I wait all the day. (Psalm 25:5 KJV)

Answer this question throughout the day:
How do I learn to walk in truth?

Pray this prayer:
Dear heavenly Father, I need help with walking out this relearning thing. Holy Spirit, please come alongside of me and help me to guard my mouth. Lead me in Your truth and teach me Your truthful ways.

Fast Answers by Beyr Reyes

Day 5

Meditate on God's Word:
Sarah was afraid, so she lied and said, "I did not laugh." But he [the Angel of the LORD] said, "Yes, you did laugh." (Genesis 18:15 NIV, author's addition in brackets)

Answer this question throughout the day:
What is the real reason I lied or continue to lie?

Pray this prayer:
Dear heavenly Father, I'm not fooling anyone. There is a reason that I lie. Many times the lie is born out of an emotion such as fear. Holy Spirit, please help me to identify and deal with the root of my lying problem.

Day 6

Meditate on God's Word:
This observance will be for you like a sign on your hand and a reminder on your forehead that this law of the LORD is to be on your lips. For the LORD brought you out of Egypt with his mighty hand. (Exodus 13:9 NIV)

Answer this question throughout the day:
When I remember my lies, what will I say about them?

Pray this prayer:
Dear heavenly Father, there is no doubt that I will be reminded of the lies I've told, and when I am, I want to use every opportunity to put Your Word on my lips. I will speak in love and truth. I will tell others of Your great love and mercy.

DAY 7

Meditate on God's Word:
Be diligent to present yourself approved to God, a worker who does not need to be ashamed, rightly dividing the word of truth. (2 Timothy 2:15 NKJV)

Answer this question throughout the day:
Will I commit to start rightly handling truth?

Pray this prayer:
Dear heavenly Father, I want to be set free from the spirit of lying. Please help me to identify the root of my lying problem. I want to present myself approved to You. Holy Spirit, please lead me in Your truthful ways and help me to retrain my mouth. When I am reminded of the times I lied, I put Your Word on my lips and speak only what is righteous. Living a life of truth will set me free, so today I will start rightly handling truth.

Fast Answers by Beyr Reyes

When You've Forsaken Someone

God understands what betrayal is. He experiences it daily. We betray Him with our rejection, we ignore His commandments, and we so easily and quickly forget what Jesus did for us on the cross.

How similar betrayal is for us. People betray other people the same way they do with God: by renouncing their love, abandoning their covenants, forgetting the good times. Generally, if someone forsakes one person, then they probably are in the habit of forsaking many.

The good news is that God *never* forsakes us. No matter how wiped out we are, He is still there to pick us up. If we just remember to keep His precepts, He will make us an eternal excellence and create a joy in us that's inextinguishable by our circumstances.

Proclamation of Fast

During this fast, I avow to:

- recognize everyone whom I have forsaken.
- confess the times I've forsaken God and His commandments.
- spend more energy telling others about God's mercy instead of justifying my actions.

Fast Answers by Beyr Reyes

When You've Forsaken Someone
1-Day Plan

Meditate on God's Word:
Even when I am old and gray, do not forsake me, my God, till I declare your power to the next generation, your mighty acts to all who are to come. (Psalm 71:18 NIV)

Answer this question throughout the day:
Do I spend more time defending my actions or telling others about God's mercy?

Pray this prayer:
Dear heavenly Father, I have forsaken friends, family, people depending on me, and leaders over me. I confess that I've even forsaken You, Father, and Your commandments. Oftentimes I try to explain and justify my actions, all to no avail. Holy Spirit, please help me to seek forgiveness and make amends. Thank You, Lord, for *never* forsaking me regardless of my pretenses. From now on, I will spend my words and time telling others of Your mercy and grace.

Fast Answers by Beyr Reyes

When You've Forsaken Someone
3-Day Plan

Day 1

Meditate on God's Word:
All the brothers of the poor hate him; how much more do his friends go far from him! He may pursue them with words, yet they abandon him. (Proverbs 19:7 NKJV)

Answer this question throughout the day:
Whom have I forsaken?

Pray this prayer:
Dear heavenly Father, my heart aches for the times I've forsaken my family and friends. There are so many times I want to go back and change the way I reacted in times of need. Lord, I regret forsaking others when they were depending on me. Your Word says that You place authorities over us and we are to support them, especially with our prayers. Lord, there have been times when I've forsaken leaders who are over me. I realize now that I was forsaking Your plan for me at that time. Father, please forgive me and help me to submit to Your plan. Holy Spirit, please help me to make a stand and never leave those in need ever again. Help me to repair all my broken relationships.

Day 2

Meditate on God's Word:
Yet ye have forsaken me, and served other gods: wherefore I will deliver you no more. (Judges 10:13 KJV)

Answer this question throughout the day:
How have I forsaken God and His Word?

Pray this prayer:
Dear heavenly Father, it's so hard for me to face the reality that I have forsaken the King of all kings and the Lord of all lords. Oftentimes when I'm lost in daily routine, I so easily and quickly forget what Jesus did for me on the cross. You know I have fallen short on Your first commandment by forsaking You. However, I have failed to meet the other nine commandments as well. I have murdered others with my words, chosen things over You, stolen, and so forth. Lord, please forgive me for forsaking Your commandments and Your Word.

DAY 3

Meditate on God's Word:
Even when I am old and gray, do not forsake me, my God, till I declare your power to the next generation, your mighty acts to all who are to come. (Psalm 71:18 NIV)

Answer this question throughout the day:
Do I spend more time defending my actions or telling others about God's mercy?

Pray this prayer:
Dear heavenly Father, I have forsaken friends, family, people depending on me, and leaders over me. I confess that I've even forsaken You, Father, and Your commandments. Oftentimes I try to explain and justify my actions, all to no avail. Holy Spirit, please help me to seek forgiveness and to make amends. Thank You, Lord, for *never* forsaking me regardless of my pretenses. From now on, I will spend my words and time telling others of Your mercy and grace.

Fast Answers by Beyr Reyes

When You've Forsaken Someone
7-Day Plan

DAY 1

Meditate on God's Word:
All the brothers of the poor hate him; how much more do his friends go far from him! He may pursue them with words, yet they abandon him. (Proverbs 19:7 NKJV)

Answer this question throughout the day:
Have I forsaken my family?

Pray this prayer:
Dear heavenly Father, my heart aches for the times when I've forsaken my family and friends. No matter how much I try to explain myself, words don't help. Holy Spirit, please help me to seek their forgiveness and make amends.

DAY 2

Meditate on God's Word:
And when all the men of Israel that were in the valley saw that they fled, and that Saul and his sons were dead, then they forsook their cities, and fled: and the Philistines came and dwelt in them. (1 Chronicles 10:7 KJV)

Answer this question throughout the day:
Have I forsaken someone who depends on me?

Pray this prayer:
Dear heavenly Father, there are so many times when I want to go back and change the way I reacted in times of need. Lord, I regret forsaking others when they were depending on me. Holy Spirit, please help me to make a

stand and to never leave those in need again. Also, please help me to repair my broken relationships.

DAY 3

Meditate on God's Word:
"But all this was done that the Scriptures of the prophets might be fulfilled." Then all the disciples forsook Him [Jesus] and fled. (Matthew 26:56 NKJV, author's additions in brackets)

Answer this question throughout the day:
Have I forsaken a leader?

Pray this prayer:
Dear heavenly Father, Your Word says that You place authorities over us and we are to support them, especially with our prayers. Lord, there have been times when I've forsaken leaders who are over me. I realize now that I was forsaking Your plan for me at that time. Father, please forgive me and help me to submit to Your will for my life.

DAY 4

Meditate on God's Word:
Yet ye have forsaken me, and served other gods: wherefore I will deliver you no more. (Judges 10:13 KJV)

Answer this question throughout the day:
Have I forsaken God?

Pray this prayer:
Dear heavenly Father, it's so hard for me to face the reality that I have forsaken the King of all kings and the Lord of all lords. Oftentimes when I'm lost in daily

routine, I so easily and quickly forget what Jesus did for me on the cross. Please forgive me and lead me to opportunities where I can share my testimony of Your great love and mercy.

Day 5

Meditate on God's Word:
And now, O our God, what shall we say after this? for we have forsaken thy commandments. (Ezra 9:10 KJV)

Answer this question throughout the day:
Have I forsaken God's Word?

Pray this prayer:
Dear heavenly Father, You know I have fallen short on Your first commandment by forsaking You. However, I have failed to meet the other nine commandments as well. I have murdered others with my words, chosen things over You, stolen, and so forth. Lord, please forgive me for forsaking Your commandments and Your Word.

Day 6

Meditate on God's Word:
For the LORD will not reject his people; he will never forsake his inheritance. (Psalm 94:14 NIV)

Answer this question throughout the day:
Who will *never* forsake me?

Pray this prayer:
Thank You, heavenly Father, that You will *never* forsake me.

DAY 7

Meditate on God's Word:
Even when I am old and gray, do not forsake me, my God, till I declare your power to the next generation, your mighty acts to all who are to come. (Psalm 71:18 NIV)

Answer this question throughout the day:
Do I spend more time defending my actions or telling others about God's mercy?

Pray this prayer:
Dear heavenly Father, I have forsaken friends, family, people depending on me, and leaders over me. I confess that I've even forsaken You, Father, and Your commandments. Oftentimes I try to explain and justify my actions, all to no avail. Holy Spirit, please help me to seek forgiveness and make amends. Thank You, Lord, for *never* forsaking me regardless of my pretenses. From now on, I will spend my words and time telling others of Your mercy and grace.

When You Need Answers and Direction

*This is what the L<small>ORD</small> says:
Stand at the crossroads and look; ask for the ancient paths, ask where the good way is, and walk in it, and you will find rest for your souls.*
(Jeremiah 6:16 <small>NIV</small>)

Fast Answers by Beyr Reyes

When You Need a Word from God

When we think about someone wanting a word from the Lord, the story of Balaam may come to mind. Balak (the king of Moab at that time) asked Balaam (a prophet) to curse the Israelites, and he offered him money to do so. Even though Balaam knew he shouldn't take the offer, he sought the Lord for an answer. Of course, when the answer was not the one Balaam wanted, he continued to ask God over and over again. Like Balaam, how many times do we keep seeking God when we already know the answer?

Sometimes we truly need to hear from the Lord on a matter. Praise God that He has given us proven methods to hear His voice. All we need to do is be open to His ways and stop trying to find answers in the world's systems.

Proclamation of Fast

During this fast, I avow to:

- seek answers through God's ordained ways.
- stop trying to find answers in the world's systems.
- listen even if the answer comes to me in a way unfamiliar to me, yet in accordance to God's Word, while keeping an open mind and heart.

Fast Answers by Beyr Reyes

When You Need a Word from God
1-Day Plan

Meditate on God's Word:
In the Law it is written: *"With other tongues and through the lips of foreigners I will speak to this people, but even then they will not listen to me, says the* LORD.*"* (1 Corinthians 14:21 NIV)

Answer this question throughout the day:
Am I really open to hearing God?

Pray this prayer:
Dear heavenly Father, please forgive me for thinking the only way that You speak is by audible voice. I understand that You use many means for speaking to us because we are not always open to just one. I will look for You to speak in Your Word, through godly people, in dreams, and through my circumstances. Lord, I will stop trying to find answers in the world's systems. I will listen, even if the answer comes to me in a way unfamiliar to me, yet in accordance to Your Word. I will keep an open mind and heart.

Fast Answers by Beyr Reyes

When You Need a Word from God
3-Day Plan

DAY 1

Meditate on God's Word:
But He answered and said, "It is written, 'Man shall not live by bread alone, but by every word that proceeds from the mouth of God.'" (Matthew 4:4 NKJV)

Answer this question throughout the day:
Where should I be looking for my answer?

Pray this prayer:
Dear heavenly Father, thank You for Your Word. I know that every page in the Bible has an answer to my question. Holy Spirit, please open my mind and heart to see what it says. Thank You for placing godly people in my life. Lord, I pray that when they speak Your will into my life that I will listen with an attentive ear and heart. Thank You for all the stories in the Bible of how You speak to people through dreams. Lord, I know that You are the same yesterday, today, and forevermore. If You used dreams then, then You will do it now. Lord, please speak to me in dreams and send me someone who can help me to interpret them. Holy Spirit, please forgive me when my doubt quenches Your voice. Please help me to keep a wide-open mind to the ways in which You speak.

DAY 2

Meditate on God's Word:
When Saul saw the Philistine army, he was afraid; terror filled his heart. He inquired of the LORD, but the LORD did not answer him by dreams or Urim or prophets. Saul then said to his attendants, "Find me a woman who is a

medium, so I may go and inquire of her." (1 Samuel 28:5–7 NIV)

Answer this question throughout the day:
Where should I *not* be looking for answers?

Pray this prayer:
Dear heavenly Father, please forgive me for looking for my answers in all the wrong places, such as horoscopes, palm readers, or other worldly venues. I will cast off these idols and turn to them no more. I will not seek wisdom from where the world seeks it. Lord, I read how You spoke to Job through a storm, so I ask that, Holy Spirit, You would keep my circumstances from blinding me, that I don't look to them and see only questions.

DAY 3

Meditate on God's Word:
In the Law it is written: "With other tongues and through the lips of foreigners I will speak to this people, but even then they will not listen to me, says the Lord." (1 Corinthians 14:21 NIV)

Answer this question throughout the day:
Am I really open to hearing God?

Pray this prayer:
Dear heavenly Father, please forgive me for thinking the only way You speak is by audible voice. I understand that You use many means for speaking to us because we are not always open to just one. I will look for You to speak in Your Word, through godly people, in dreams, and through my circumstances. Lord, I will stop trying to find answers in the world's systems. I will listen even if the answer comes to me in a way that is unfamiliar to me, yet in accordance to Your Word. I will keep an open mind and heart.

Fast Answers by Beyr Reyes

When You Need a Word from God
7-Day Plan

DAY 1

Meditate on God's Word:
But He answered and said, "It is written, 'Man shall not live by bread alone, but by every word that proceeds from the mouth of God.'" (Matthew 4:4 NKJV)

Answer this question throughout the day:
Am I searching God's Word for my answer?

Pray this prayer:
Dear heavenly Father, thank You for Your Word. I know that every page in the Bible has an answer to my question. Holy Spirit, please open my mind and heart to see what it says. Lord, please speak to me through Your Word.

DAY 2

Meditate on God's Word:
For this reason we also thank God without ceasing, because when you received the word of God which you heard from us, you welcomed it not as the word of men, but as it is in truth, the word of God, which also effectively works in you who believe. (1 Thessalonians 2:13 NKJV)

Answer this question throughout the day:
Am I listening for God to speak through others?

Pray this prayer:
Dear heavenly Father, thank You for placing godly people in my life. Lord, I pray that when they speak

Your will into my life that I will listen with an attentive ear and heart. Holy Spirit, please lead me into discernment.

DAY 3

Meditate on God's Word:
But when he, the Spirit of truth, comes, he will guide you into all the truth. He will not speak on his own; he will speak only what he hears, and he will tell you what is yet to come. (John 16:13 NIV)

Answer this question throughout the day:
Am I allowing the Holy Spirit to speak?

Pray this prayer:
Dear heavenly Father, thank You for the Spirit of truth. Holy Spirit, please forgive me when my doubt quenches Your voice. Please help me to keep a wide-open mind to the ways in which You speak.

DAY 4

Meditate on God's Word:
The angel of God said to me in the dream, "Jacob." I answered, "Here I am." (Genesis 31:11 NIV)

Answer this question throughout the day:
Am I open to hearing from God through dreams?

Pray this prayer:
Dear heavenly Father, thank You for all the stories in the Bible of how You speak to people through dreams. Lord, I know that You are the same yesterday, today, and forevermore. If You used dreams then, then You will do it now. Please forgive me for letting the enemy trick me into thinking dreams are evil and just part of other religions. I recognize that the enemy perverted the perception of this

awesome tool You created for communication with us. Lord, please speak to me in dreams and send me someone who can help me to interpret them.

Day 5

Meditate on God's Word:
When Saul saw the Philistine army, he was afraid; terror filled his heart. He inquired of the LORD, but the LORD did not answer him by dreams or Urim or prophets. Saul then said to his attendants, "Find me a woman who is a medium, so I may go and inquire of her." (1 Samuel 28:5–7 NIV)

Answer this question throughout the day:
Am I looking to horoscopes, palm readers, or other worldly venues for my answers?

Pray this prayer:
Dear heavenly Father, please forgive me for looking for my answers in all the wrong places. I will cast off these idols and turn to them no more. I will not seek wisdom from where the world seeks it.

Day 6

Meditate on God's Word:
Then the LORD spoke to Job out of the storm. (Job 38:1 NIV)

Answer this question throughout the day:
Can God speak to me through my circumstances?

Pray this prayer:
Dear heavenly Father, I read how You spoke to Job through a storm, so I ask that You speak to me out of

mine. Lord, please use my circumstances as a means of getting Your message through to me. Holy Spirit, I pray that You keep my circumstances from blinding me.

DAY 7

Meditate on God's Word:
In the Law it is written: "With other tongues and through the lips of foreigners I will speak to this people, but even then they will not listen to me, says the Lord." (1 Corinthians 14:21 NIV)

Answer this question throughout the day:
Am I really open to hearing God?

Pray this prayer:
Dear heavenly Father, please forgive me for thinking the only way You speak is by audible voice. I understand that You use many means for speaking to us because we are not always open to just one. I will look for You to speak in Your Word, through godly people, in dreams, and through my circumstances. Lord, I will stop trying to find answers in the world's systems. I will listen even if the answer comes to me in a way unfamiliar to me, yet in accordance to Your Word. I will keep an open mind and heart.

Fast Answers by Beyr Reyes

When You Need a New Mindset and Way of Thinking

Sometime we get stuck in a rut. Oftentimes, the rut is nothing more than a dysfunctional mindset and a crippled way of thinking.

In the book of Romans, the Bible says that we can be transformed by the renewing of our minds. When this happens, we are then able to understand what God's will is and walk in the plan He has for our life. Having this new mindset is not the end, though. We must protect it daily and be on guard against the enemy who comes to kill, steal, and destroy it and us.

Proclamation of Fast

During this fast, I avow to:

- come to the full understanding of who I am in Christ.
- use my new point of view to walk in the fantastic plan God has for my life.
- put on the full armor of God to protect this new mindset.

Fast Answers by Beyr Reyes

When You Need a New Mindset and Way of Thinking
1-Day Plan

Meditate on God's Word:
Stand therefore, having girded your waist with truth, having put on the breastplate of righteousness, and having shod your feet with the preparation of the gospel of peace; above all, taking the shield of faith with which you will be able to quench all the fiery darts of the wicked one. And take the helmet of salvation, and the sword of the Spirit, which is the word of God. (Ephesians 6:14–17 NKJV)

Answer this question throughout the day:
What am I willing to do to get a new mindset and keep it?

Pray this prayer:
Dear heavenly Father, thank You for showing me who I really am—a child of the King, fearfully and wonderfully made. I am a new creature, in which there is *no* condemnation. Lord, You have a fantastic plan for my life, and I will use my new point of view to walk in it. Thank You for giving me a new outlook. I will put on the full armor of God to protect this new mindset.

Fast Answers by Beyr Reyes

When You Need a New Mindset and Way of Thinking
3-Day Plan

DAY 1

Meditate on God's Word:
Therefore if any man be in Christ, he is a new creature: old things are passed away; behold, all things are become new. (2 Corinthians 5:17 KJV)

Answer this question throughout the day:
Am I the same person I used to be?

Pray this prayer:
Dear heavenly Father, thank You for loving me enough to make me like no other and for giving me a purpose that no other can fulfill. Holy Spirit, please help me to destroy the low self-esteem that challenges my belief that I am wonderfully made. Father, thank You for not condemning me, and please help me to stop condemning myself. Thank You for my new life in Jesus Christ. You have made me new. I refuse to return to my old self. Thank You, God, that I'm not who I used to be. All bad habits, addictions, and lousy attitudes are passed away. Lord, please help me to wrap my head around the fact that I'm the son/daughter of the King and to realize my rights and privileges of this royalty. Just as we see the families of earthly kings being healthy, wealthy, and wise, I, too, will accept this blessing in my own life. I will act according to Your Kingdom principles.

DAY 2

Meditate on God's Word:
For I know the thoughts that I think toward you, says the LORD, *thoughts of peace and not of evil, to give*

you a future and a hope. (Jeremiah 29:11 NKJV)

Answer this question throughout the day:
What kind of plan does God have for my life?

Pray this prayer:
Dear heavenly Father, please help me to change my point of view. No longer do I want to be doubting, suspicious, and negative all the time. Lord, Your Word says that whatever we think on, we become. Instead of considering the impossible, I will see possibilities. Instead of seeing death, I will see life. Thank You, Father, for Your plan for my life. Your Word says that You knew me even in the womb, even before You formed me. I want to walk in Your will and not get in the way of Your intentions for me. I want what You have for me.

DAY 3

Meditate on God's Word:
Stand therefore, having girded your waist with truth, having put on the breastplate of righteousness, and having shod your feet with the preparation of the gospel of peace; above all, taking the shield of faith with which you will be able to quench all the fiery darts of the wicked one. And take the helmet of salvation, and the sword of the Spirit, which is the word of God. (Ephesians 6:14–17 NKJV)

Answer this question throughout the day:
What am I willing to do to protect my thoughts?

Pray this prayer:
Dear heavenly Father, thank You for showing me who I really am—a child of the King, fearfully and wonderfully made. I am a new creature, in which there is *no* condemnation. Lord, You have a fantastic plan for my life, and I will use my new point of view to walk in it. Thank You for giving me a new outlook. I will put on the full armor of God to protect this new mindset.

Fast Answers by Beyr Reyes

When You Need a New Mindset and Way of Thinking
7-Day Plan

DAY 1

Meditate on God's Word:
I will praise thee; for I am fearfully and wonderfully made: marvellous are thy works; and that my soul knoweth right well. (Psalm 139:14 KJV)

Answer this question throughout the day:
Do I really think that I am fearfully and wonderfully made?

Pray this prayer:
Dear heavenly Father, thank You for loving me enough to make me like no other and for giving me a purpose that no other can fulfill. Holy Spirit, please help me to destroy the low self-esteem that challenges my belief that I am wonderfully made.

DAY 2

Meditate on God's Word:
There is therefore now no condemnation to them which are in Christ Jesus, who walk not after the flesh, but after the Spirit. (Romans 8:1 KJV)

Answer this question throughout the day:
Who is condemning me?

Pray this prayer:
Dear heavenly Father, thank You for not condemning me, and please help me to stop condemning myself.

Fast Answers by Beyr Reyes

DAY 3

Meditate on God's Word:
Therefore if any man be in Christ, he is a new creature: old things are passed away; behold, all things are become new. (2 Corinthians 5:17 KJV)

Answer this question throughout the day:
Am I the same person I used to be?

Pray this prayer:
Dear heavenly Father, thank You for my new life in Jesus Christ. You have made me new, and I refuse to return to my old self. Thank You, God, that I'm not who I used to be. All bad habits, addictions, and lousy attitudes are passed away.

DAY 4

Meditate on God's Word:
See what great love the Father has lavished on us, that we should be called children of God! And that is what we are! (1 John 3:1 NIV)

Answer this question throughout the day:
Do I act like a child of the King?

Pray this prayer:
Dear heavenly Father, please help me to wrap my head around the fact that I'm the son/daughter of the King. I am royalty. Please help me realize my rights and privileges of this royalty. Just as we see the families of earthly kings being healthy, wealthy, and wise, I, too, will accept this blessing in my own life. I will act according to Your Kingdom principles.

Fast Answers by Beyr Reyes

Day 5

Meditate on God's Word:
Finally, brothers and sisters, whatever is true, whatever is noble, whatever is right, whatever is pure, whatever is lovely, whatever is admirable—if anything is excellent or praiseworthy—think about such things. (Philippians 4:8 NIV)

Answer this question throughout the day:
What do I spend most of my time thinking about?

Pray this prayer:
Dear heavenly Father, please help me to change my point of view. No longer do I want to be doubting, suspicious, and negative all the time. Lord, Your Word says that whatever we think on, we become. Holy Spirit, please help me to change my mindset. Instead of considering the impossible, I will see possibilities. Instead of seeing death, I will see life.

Day 6

Meditate on God's Word:
For I know the thoughts that I think toward you, says the LORD, thoughts of peace and not of evil, to give you a future and a hope. (Jeremiah 29:11 NKJV)

Answer this question throughout the day:
What kind of plan does God have for my life?

Pray this prayer:
Dear heavenly Father, thank You for Your plan for my life. Your Word says that You knew me even in the womb, even before You formed me. I want to walk in Your will and not get in the way of Your intentions for me. I want what You have for me.

Fast Answers by Beyr Reyes

DAY 7

Meditate on God's Word:
Stand therefore, having girded your waist with truth, having put on the breastplate of righteousness, and having shod your feet with the preparation of the gospel of peace; above all, taking the shield of faith with which you will be able to quench all the fiery darts of the wicked one. And take the helmet of salvation, and the sword of the Spirit, which is the word of God. (Ephesians 6:14–17 NKJV)

Answer this question throughout the day:
What am I willing to do to protect my thoughts?

Pray this prayer:
Dear heavenly Father, thank You for showing me who I really am—a child of the King, fearfully and wonderfully made. I am a new creature, in which there is *no* condemnation. Lord, You have a fantastic plan for my life, and I will use my new point of view to walk in it. Thank You for giving me a new outlook. I will put on the full armor of God to protect this new mindset.

Fast Answers by Beyr Reyes

When You Need Confirmation

The Bible says that the ears test words as the tongue tastes food. This couldn't be any more true. How many times do we decide whether to accept something based on how well it pleases us?

Confirmation is a godly thing. Several time in the Scriptures, God confirmed a word that was sent forth or a covenant that He made. We, too, should follow this example. We need to be careful not to swallow everything hanging in front of us. Just ask your local fish and it will agree.

Proclamation of Fast

During this fast, I avow to:

- look for confirmation through signs and wonders, written or spoken decrees, witnesses, and the Holy Spirit.
- test all answers and confirmations against the Word of God.
- be open to hearing from God regardless of the method He chooses to communicate.

Fast Answers by Beyr Reyes

When You Need Confirmation
1-Day Plan

Meditate on God's Word:
The hearing ear and the seeing eye, the LORD has made them both. (Proverbs 20:12 NKJV)

Answer this question throughout the day:
Am I really open to hearing from God?

Pray this prayer:
Dear heavenly Father, thank You that You always send confirmation for the answers You provide. Please help me to accept Your different methods, such as signs and wonders, written or spoken decrees, witnesses, and of course, the Holy Spirit. I will test all answers and confirmations against Your Word to see whether they are good and of Your will for me. Please help me to refrain from hearing things that just tickle my ears. Lord, I want to be open to hearing from You. I want eyes to see and ears to hear.

Fast Answers by Beyr Reyes

When You Need Confirmation
3-Day Plan

Day 1

Meditate on God's Word:
I speak the truth in Christ—I am not lying, my conscience confirms it through the Holy Spirit. (Romans 9:1 NIV)

Answer this question throughout the day:
Is God speaking to me through methods that I may have overlooked as coincidences?

Pray this prayer:
Dear heavenly Father, thank You for Your Holy Spirit, who confirms Your will for my life. Please help my mind and heart to be open to what the Spirit says. Please send me signs and wonders to confirm my answers. I will not overlook even the smallest one as a coincidence. Father, please open my eyes to any decrees that You have sent for my confirmation. I will look for them in the form of announcements, rulings, declarations, proclamations, etc. Please confirm Your answer to me out of the mouths of two or three witnesses. Lord, I understand that You will speak through a TV person just as well as a person face-to-face. Lord, if I already failed to catch any confirmations, please remind me.

Day 2

Meditate on God's Word:
Do not quench the Spirit. Do not despise prophecies. Test all things; hold fast what is good. (1 Thessalonians 5:19–21 NKJV)

Fast Answers by Beyr Reyes

Answer this question throughout the day:
Do I take the time to test the word I get against God's Word?

Pray this prayer:
Dear heavenly Father, thank You for the times when Your answers come slowly and allow us a chance to align our thoughts and minds. Lord, thank You, too, for fast answers that keep us from having to wait. Regardless of the speed, I will take the time to test *all* answers against Your Word.

DAY 3

Meditate on God's Word:
The hearing ear and the seeing eye, the LORD *has made them both.* (Proverbs 20:12 NKJV)

Answer this question throughout the day:
Am I really open to hearing from God?

Pray this prayer:
Dear heavenly Father, thank You that You always send confirmation for the answers You provide. Please help me to accept Your different methods, such as signs and wonders, written or spoken decrees, witnesses, and of course, the Holy Spirit. I will test all answers and confirmations against Your Word to see whether they are good and of Your will for me. Please help me to refrain from hearing things that just tickle my ears. Lord, I want to be open to hearing from You. I want eyes to see and ears to hear.

Fast Answers by Beyr Reyes

When You Need Confirmation
7-Day Plan

Day 1

Meditate on God's Word:
I speak the truth in Christ—I am not lying, my conscience confirms it through the Holy Spirit. (Romans 9:1 NIV)

Answer this question throughout the day:
What does my spirit say?

Pray this prayer:
Dear heavenly Father, thank You for Your Holy Spirit, who confirms Your will for my life. Please help my mind and heart to be open to what the Spirit says.

Day 2

Meditate on God's Word:
Do not quench the Spirit. Do not despise prophecies. Test all things; hold fast what is good. (1 Thessalonians 5 NKJV)

Answer this question throughout the day:
Do I take the time to test the word I get against God's Word?

Pray this prayer:
Dear heavenly Father, thank You for the times when Your answers come slowly and allow us a chance to align our thoughts and minds. Lord, thank You, too, for fast answers that keep us from having to wait. Regardless of the speed, I will take the time to test *all* answers against Your Word.

Fast Answers by Beyr Reyes

DAY 3

Meditate on God's Word:
So Paul and Barnabas spent considerable time there, speaking boldly for the Lord, who confirmed the message of his grace by enabling them to perform signs and wonders. (Acts 14:3 NIV)

Answer this question throughout the day:
Is God speaking to me through signs and wonders that I may have overlooked as coincidences?

Pray this prayer:
Dear heavenly Father, please send me signs and wonders to confirm my answers. I will not overlook even the smallest one as a coincidence. Lord, I understand that You will speak through a TV person just as well as a person face-to-face.

DAY 4

Meditate on God's Word:
And the decree of Esther confirmed these matters of Purim; and it was written in the book. (Esther 9:32 KJV)

Answer this question throughout the day:
Have I witnessed a written or spoken decree that confirms?

Pray this prayer:
Dear heavenly Father, please open my eyes to any decrees that You have sent for my confirmation. I will look for them in the form of announcements, rulings, declarations, proclamations, etc.

Fast Answers by Beyr Reyes

DAY 5

Meditate on God's Word:
This will be my third visit to you. "Every matter must be established by the testimony of two or three witnesses." (2 Corinthians 13:1 NIV)

Answer this question throughout the day:
How many confirmations have I received?

Pray this prayer:
Dear heavenly Father, please confirm Your answer through two or three ways to me. Lord, if I already failed to catch them, please remind me.

DAY 6

Meditate on God's Word:
For the time will come when they will not endure sound doctrine, but according to their own desires, because they have itching ears, they will heap up for themselves teachers; and they will turn their ears away from the truth, and be turned aside to fables. (2 Timothy 4:3–4 NKJV)

Answer this question throughout the day:
Am I hearing what I want to hear and not what God wants me to hear?

Pray this prayer:
Dear heavenly Father, please forgive me if You have already answered and confirmed my question, and yet I failed to acknowledge it. Sometimes I turn off godly answers that go against my fleshly desires. Holy Spirit, please help me not to hear only what I want to hear.

Day 7

Meditate on God's Word:
The hearing ear and the seeing eye, the LORD has made them both. (Proverbs 20:12 NKJV)

Answer this question throughout the day:
Am I really open to hearing from God?

Pray this prayer:
Dear heavenly Father, thank You that You always send confirmation for the answers You provide. Please help me to accept Your different methods, such as signs and wonders, written or spoken decrees, witnesses, and of course, the Holy Spirit. I will test all answers and confirmations against Your Word to see whether they are good and of Your will for me. Please help me to refrain from hearing things that just tickle my ears. Lord, I want to be open to hearing from You. I want eyes to see and ears to hear.

Fast Answers by Beyr Reyes

When You Want God's Will for Your Life

Jesus is our example of Someone who truly wanted the Father's will for His life. While Jesus was praying in the Garden, the sins of the world were being laid upon Him. Let's just stop a minute to reflect on the magnitude of this event. Imagine how we feel when we know we've really sinned in a big way. Now multiply that by every sin we've ever committed and then multiply that by every person who has, or who will ever, live on earth. Jesus was so overcome that He said, "My soul is exceedingly sorrowful, even to death" (Mark 14:34 NKJV).

What was Jesus' response during this misery? He cried out to the Father and said, "Not My will, but Yours." Simply amazing.

If we ever want to hear the Lord tell us, "Well done, My good and faithful servant," then we need to get on the right path—His path.

Proclamation of Fast

During this fast, I avow to:

- learn to do the will of God.
- recognize that God's will is for us here on earth.
- submit to God's will.

Fast Answers by Beyr Reyes

When You Want God's Will for Your Life
1-Day Plan

Meditate on God's Word:
And he said unto them, Go ye into all the world, and preach the gospel to every creature. (Mark 16:15 KJV)

Answer this question throughout the day:
What was the last directive Jesus gave us before He ascended into heaven?

Pray this prayer:
Dear heavenly Father, please teach me to do Your will, even if I must relearn some things. Lord, I know You have a plan for my life, not just in heaven, but while I'm here on earth, too. I desire Your ways and submit to them. Father, I know Your ultimate will is for all to be saved. Holy Spirit, please help me to share the Gospel. Please present me with opportunities to tell others of Your saving grace and mercies.

Fast Answers by Beyr Reyes

When You Want God's Will for Your Life
3-Day Plan

DAY 1

Meditate on God's Word:
Teach me to do Your will, for You are my God; Your Spirit is good. Lead me in the land of uprightness. (Psalm 143:10 NKJV)

Answer this question throughout the day:
Am I willing to relearn some things?

Pray this prayer:
Dear heavenly Father, I desire Your will for my life, and I understand that it may be in direct contrast to the ways I currently live and think. Holy Spirit, please help me to relearn Your ways. Lord, please teach me to do Your will.

DAY 2

Meditate on God's Word:
Thy kingdom come, Thy will be done in earth, as it is in heaven. (Matthew 6:10 KJV)

Answer this question throughout the day:
Are all God's plans for my future tied to eternity, or is it His will to prosper me on earth?

Pray this prayer:
Dear heavenly Father, thank You for Your plan for my life. Your Word says that You knew me even in the womb, even before You formed me. I want to walk in Your will and not get in the way of Your intentions for me. I want what You have for me. Jesus said that He will give us the keys of the Kingdom, and that anything we bind on earth

will be bound in heaven, and whatever we loose on earth will be loosed in heaven. His words make it clear that we can have eternal blessings while we are still on the earth. Thank You, Jesus, for confirming this to me in the Lord's Prayer, which You gave the disciples to teach them how to pray.

Day 3

Meditate on God's Word:
And he said unto them, Go ye into all the world, and preach the gospel to every creature. (Mark 16:15 KJV)

Answer this question throughout the day:
What was the last directive Jesus gave us before He ascended into heaven?

Pray this prayer:
Dear heavenly Father, please teach me to do Your will, even if I must relearn some things. Lord, I know You have a plan for my life, not just in heaven, but while I'm here on earth, too. I desire Your ways and submit to them. Father, I know Your ultimate will is for all to be saved. Holy Spirit, please help me to share the Gospel. Please present me with opportunities to tell others of Your saving grace and mercies.

Fast Answers by Beyr Reyes

When You Want God's Will for Your Life
7-Day Plan

DAY 1

Meditate on God's Word:
Teach me to do Your will, for You are my God; Your Spirit is good. Lead me in the land of uprightness. (Psalm 143:10 NKJV)

Answer this question throughout the day:
Am I willing to relearn some things?

Pray this prayer:
Dear heavenly Father, I desire Your will for my life, and I understand that it may be in direct contrast to the ways I currently live and think. Holy Spirit, please help me to relearn Your ways. Lord, please teach me to do Your will.

DAY 2

Meditate on God's Word:
For I know the thoughts that I think toward you, says the LORD, thoughts of peace and not of evil, to give you a future and a hope. (Jeremiah 29:11 NKJV)

Answer this question throughout the day:
What is God's plan for my life?

Pray this prayer:
Dear heavenly Father, thank You for Your plan for my life. Your Word says that You knew me even in the womb, even before You formed me. I want to walk in Your will and not get in the way of Your intentions for me. I want what You have for me.

Day 3

Meditate on God's Word:
Thy kingdom come, Thy will be done in earth, as it is in heaven. (Matthew 6:10 KJV)

Answer this question throughout the day:
Are all God's plans for my future tied to eternity, or is it His will to prosper me on earth?

Pray this prayer:
Dear heavenly Father, Jesus said that He will give us the keys of the Kingdom, and that anything we bind on earth will be bound in heaven, and whatever we loose on earth will be loosed in heaven. His words make it clear that we can have eternal blessings while we are still on the earth. Thank You, Jesus, for confirming this to me in the Lord's Prayer, which You gave the disciples to teach them how to pray.

Day 4

Meditate on God's Word:
I desire to do your will, my God; your law is within my heart. (Psalm 40:8 NIV)

Answer this question throughout the day:
How much do I desire to do God's will?

Pray this prayer:
Dear heavenly Father, please forgive me for desiring to do Your will only until it becomes hard or uncomfortable. I want to crave and seek Your will at all times—not just when it makes me feel warm and cuddly.

Fast Answers by Beyr Reyes

Day 5

Meditate on God's Word:
For this is good and acceptable in the sight of God our Savior, who desires all men to be saved and to come to the knowledge of the truth. (1 Timothy 2:3–4 NKJV)

Answer this question throughout the day:
What is God's ultimate will for us on earth?

Pray this prayer:
Dear heavenly Father, You make it perfectly clear what Your ultimate will is for us while we are on earth. You desire for all to be saved. Holy Spirit, please help me to share my testimony and help bring others to the saving knowledge of Jesus Christ.

Day 6

Meditate on God's Word:
By myself I can do nothing; I judge only as I hear, and my judgment is just, for I seek not to please myself but him who sent me. (John 5:30 NIV)

Answer this question throughout the day:
Am I submitting to God's will or seeking another way?

Pray this prayer:
Dear heavenly Father, even Jesus submitted His life to Your will regardless of how hard it was. I want to be like Jesus, to please You and not just please myself. Holy Spirit, help me to submit to the Father's will. I refuse to keep looking around for alternative opportunities or possibilities.

DAY 7

Meditate on God's Word:
And he said unto them, Go ye into all the world, and preach the gospel to every creature. (Mark 16:15 KJV)

Answer this question throughout the day:
What was the last directive Jesus gave us before He ascended into heaven?

Pray this prayer:
Dear heavenly Father, please teach me to do Your will, even if I must relearn some things. Lord, I know You have a plan for my life, not just in heaven, but while I'm here on earth, too. I desire Your ways and submit to them. Father, I know Your ultimate will is for all to be saved. Holy Spirit, please help me to share the Gospel. Please present me with opportunities to tell others of Your saving grace and mercies.

OTHER IDEAS FOR FASTING

Fast Answers by Beyr Reyes

Scripture Fast

During a Scripture fast, a person would set aside a certain number of days to read and meditate on a piece of Scripture. For example, each day could focus on a specific Bible verse or chapter. The book of Psalms is especially well-suited for this sort of fast. Each of the psalms has elements of praise, repentance, despair, etc.; however, many are rich in certain themes, as they were written out of the heart of a psalmist in response to situations and feelings. Following is a list of examples. (Please note that this list is not exhaustive by any means, but only serves to give example of psalms that are thematic in general.)

- Praising God: Psalms 24, 65, 66, 84, 93, 96, 145, 148, 149, and 150
- Looking for God: Psalm 13
- Thankfulness: Psalm 16 and 1 Chronicles 16:7–36
- Spiritual warfare: Psalm 18
- Reassurance and peace: Psalms 23 and 139

Psalm 119 is special, in that its 176 verses are divided into twenty-two stanzas, one for each letter of the Hebrew alphabet. This psalm could be used for a twenty-two day or week fast.

Psalms 120–134 are often referred to as the Song of Ascents. Scholars theorize that as Jews made their way up the fifteen steps leading to the Hulda Gate (the main entrance of the Temple Mount), they would sing the fifteen Psalms of Ascent as they went up to worship.

Groups or Types of People

We are called to pray for groups of individuals, especially those in influential positions.

> *Therefore I exhort first of all that supplications, prayers, intercessions, and giving of thanks be made for all men, for kings and all who are in authority, that we may lead a quiet and peaceable life in all godliness and reverence.*

Fast Answers by Beyr Reyes

For this is good and acceptable in the sight of God our Savior. (1 Timothy 2:1–3 NKJV)

One way to fast for a group of people is to fast a certain amount of time (i.e., a day or week) for each one. Some groups that need our prayer include:

- Our children
- Our friends and other family members
- Local or national churches and pastors
- Elected and appointed government officials (you could fast a day each for local, state, and federal)
- Business and business leaders
- Schools, teachers, and administrators
- Judges and courts (you could fast a day each for local, state, and federal)
- Influential celebrities and spokespersons
- Troops and servicemen (you could fast a day for army, marines, navy, air force, National Guard, Coast Guard, etc.)
- Israel (Psalm 122:6 KJV: *Pray for the peace of Jerusalem: they shall prosper that love thee.*)
- Those who persecute or mistreat you (Matthew 5:44 NIV: *But I tell you, love your enemies and pray for those who persecute you*; Luke 6:28 NIV: *Bless those who curse you, pray for those who mistreat you.*)
- Missionaries
- Whomever or whatever God lays upon your heart

To Accomplish Something

Fasting to accomplish a goal or to prepare for an important milestone is common. Some of these events include:

- writing a book (like I did for this one)
- preparing for marriage

- planning an event or occasion
- preparing for a milestone in life (i.e., decade birthdays)

When You Don't Know the Reason

Sometimes we may have an inclination to fast without an obvious reason. That's okay. When we don't know what to fast for, we can simply open ourselves to the Holy Spirit according to Romans 8:26:

> *In the same way, the Spirit helps us in our weakness. We do not know what we ought to pray for, but the Spirit himself intercedes for us through wordless groans.* (NIV)

Fast Answers by Beyr Reyes

Fast Answers by Beyr Reyes

About the Author

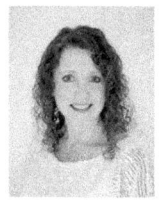

BEYR REYES received her doctorate degree in biomedical science. She has produced over 200 publications in science, medicine, and Christian genres. In addition, she has worked in the drug industry since 2005 as a regulatory writer for major pharmaceutical and biotech companies. (Beyr Reyes is Jennifer Minigh's pen name for the Christian genre.)

See Beyr's author page at
http://www.shadetreepublishing.com/beyr-reyes.html.

Author's Acknowledgments

Thank You, Lord, for pouring into me during the writing of this book.

Thank You, David and Julia, for loving me—especially during the forty-day fast when I wrote this book.

Thank you, Pastor Chuck Lawrence, for feeding my mind and spirit with God's Word. Thanks to the multitude of other pastors and ministry leaders who made their mark on my life.

Fast Answers by Beyr Reyes

Fast Answers by Beyr Reyes

See Beyr's Other Books

The Big Picture
2011 Readers' Favorite
Bronze Award

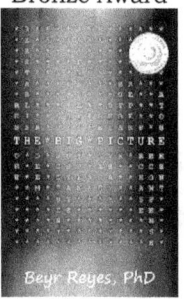

Subject Your Flesh
2014 CSPA
e-Book of the Year

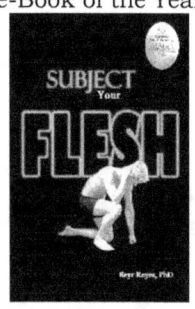

Make a Choice
2011 Readers' Favorite
Silver Award

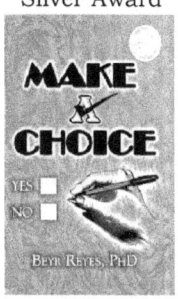

489: A Short Story About Forgiveness
2016 CSPA General Fiction Book of the Year

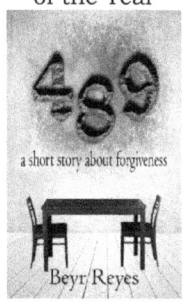

**Renewable Energy:
A Short Story About Second Chances**

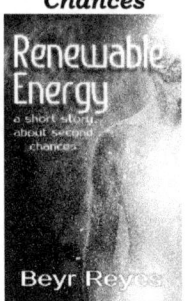

**Relaying the Word:
A 16-Week Trek Through the Bible with Friends**

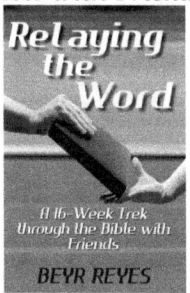

Fast Answers by Beyr Reyes

Fast Answers by Beyr Reyes

NOTES

Fast Answers by Beyr Reyes

Fast Answers by Beyr Reyes

Fast Answers by Beyr Reyes

www.ingramcontent.com/pod-product-compliance
Lightning Source LLC
Chambersburg PA
CBHW071206070526
44584CB00019B/2941